In the Frontier

What Consumers Should Know about Alternative Medicine

by Dr. Alejandro Carballo

DORRANCE
PUBLISHING CO
EST. 1920
PITTSBURGH, PENNSYLVANIA 15238

Dorrance Publishing Co
585 Alpha Drive
Pittsburgh, PA 15238
Visit our website at *www.dorrancebookstore.com*

ISBN: 978-1-6470-2503-8
eISBN: 978-1-6470-2724-7

In the Frontier

*What Consumers Should Know
about Alternative Medicine*

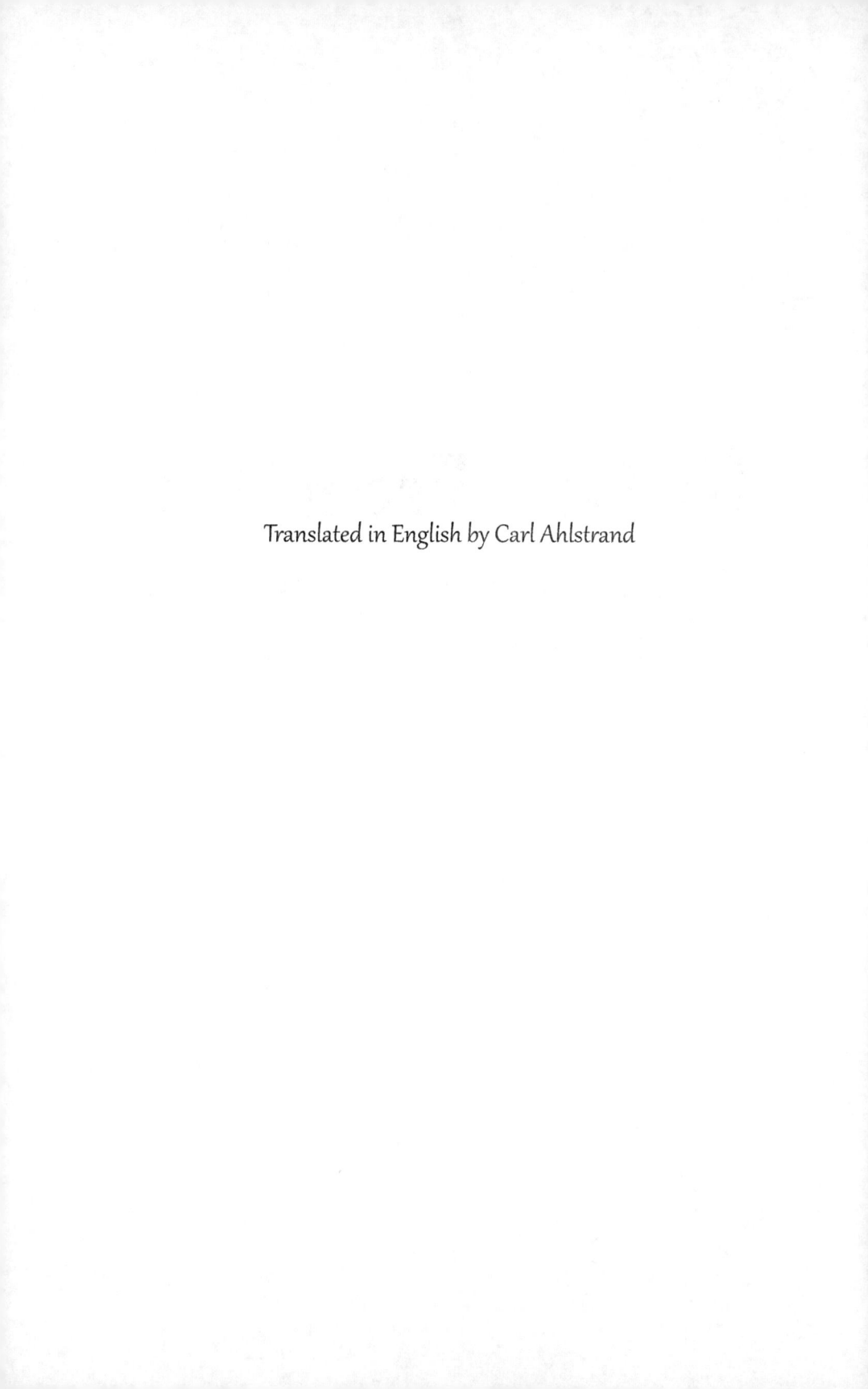

Translated in English by Carl Ahlstrand

Contents

About the Author

Alejandro Carballo is a physician with 30 years of professional experience. He is a specialist in clinical pharmacology, general medicine, and occupational health service. He has also undergone 40 years of self-study in complementary medicine.

He was born in 1960 in the Cuban capital city of Havana. Between 1985 and 1992, he was one of the leading names in the Cuban healthcare system as he led a research team tasked with developing a new healthcare system based on herbal medicine. The team produced basic research as well as clinical trials on the use of herbal medicine and complementary methods with over 60,000 patients. During this time, he also worked in the Cuban parliament and was one of the prominent figures in Cuban healthcare politics.

The research project was eventually stifled due to political pressure. Alejandro and his team were being forced to stand behind certain recommendations to the Cuban healthcare system. Alejandro felt this was in violation of human rights and he also publicly expressed those feelings, which did not sit well with the leaders. After participating in a medical convention in Stockholm in 1994, Alejandro applied for political asylum in Sweden.

In 1997, he started the first educational program in herbal and complementary medicine for medical students at Karolinska Institutet. He has also been a consultant to the Swedish Medical Products Agency about the registry of herbal medicine, and he has represented Sweden at the European Committee for Homeopathy. At present, he runs a healthcare centre and occupational health service in Sweden as well as a project, Spiragreen Sweden, committed to non-pharmaceutical health promotion and selfcare.

Alejandro Carballo is responsible for this book, the purpose of which is to inform people about the most common methods of complementary treatment. It is his hope that some of these methods will eventually become better integrated into the evidence-based healthcare system.

The official healthcare system is based on proven effectiveness. There is no "alternative" to the healthcare system that can guarantee preventive measures, correct diagnosis and treatment of diseases and their symptoms and/or complications. However, the system for assessing evidence is strongly influenced by the pharmaceutical industry's interests.

- Can some methods be a complement in the prevention and treatment of diseases and ill health?
- Is it not risky to trust in the assessment of people whose education/experience is far from that of medical personnel?
- Should you trust in methods that can be both harmful and cause a delay in the making of a correct diagnosis?

Introduction

Have you ever taken a painkiller? Most people answer yes to that question. But many shake their heads when asked the follow-up question: *Do you know how the chemical substances in the painkiller affect your body?* Why is that? Why do we not care about what happens in our bodies when we use pharmaceuticals? Many people glance at the leaflet and read, perhaps with a little amusement, that you might get a headache from the headache drug. But if you think about it, it is rather frightening. How can we stuff ourselves with preparations that can cause such dreadful side effects as diarrhoea, skin rash, contractions of the airway muscles, intestinal bleeding, and increased risk of heart attack and stroke? These are all listed side effects from one of the most common painkillers that we use almost daily. The answer to the question is that we are conditioned to trust the healthcare system and the pharmaceutical industry—for better or worse.

The art of medicine in Western culture is based on scientific research and proven effects. We call this an *evidence-based healthcare*. This contrasts with traditionally based healthcare systems, such as the traditional Chinese medicine and other Eastern medical teachings. These are instead often based on unproven theories or long experience. The evidence-based healthcare system is a product of our scientific history, and in our modern society, it is a rigorous and effective system that ensures a high-quality medical care. That is why we can trust the healthcare system, and we know that our physicians and medical staff work according to specific principles to help us in the best way possible. However, we also live in a complex world where money, power, and political agendas carry a lot of weight. It is our medical universities that, by order of the state, have the ultimate responsibility for research and development. But historically, it is the pharmaceutical industry that has financed research and development in medicine, and thus helped shape our understanding of how diseases and symptoms are prevented and treated. This means that we have been taught to trust an understanding of diseases that, in many cases, is strongly influenced by the pharmaceutical companies and their economic interests. What is your opinion on that?

A direct consequence of this is that we seem to regard our bodies as laboratories. We accept that diseases and symptoms are treated by introducing chemical products into our bodies. Granted, these products are rigorously tested, and their effects are proven, but beyond the desired result, they also have a confirmed effect on the entire body. For example, a painkiller will affect each and every cell in your body in one way or another even though its only job is to relieve pain in, say, an aching joint. As long as the active substance in a preparation has the desired effect, and as long as the mechanism behind that effect is mapped out, it does not seem to matter so much that the mechanisms behind the side effects are not thoroughly mapped out. What you do not know cannot hurt you, right? The ignorance is frightening.

Fact and truth are relative and fleeting concepts that ought to be used with greater care. The principles that today guide our approach and our understanding of how human beings are built were not the same a hundred years ago, and what is obvious to us today might well be tomorrow's greatest doubt. That is why we must dare to be critical and willing to question and re-examine "facts" all the time. Today, many of us are aware of how economic interests can trump the willingness to help people.

In recent years, the interest in alternative treatment methods has grown rapidly in the West, and it continues to grow. Exercises like yoga and qigong have become increasingly popular, and the same can be said for acupuncture, mindfulness, and breathing exercises. Health magazines, and other periodicals, too, for that matter, are brimming with tips on how you breathe away your pain or which yoga postures are best for your back pain. Up to a point, I consider this to be a good development, since many people are helped by these methods. Most of these methods have a very long history, dating back several thousand years, and they would probably not have survived into our time if they were not effective. Of course, a long history is no guarantee that something is good. Just look at smoking, for example. We humans have smoked various things in various ways for pretty much as long as we have existed. It is also important to remember to take everything with moderation and not fall for all the tips about breathing away your pain. What I am trying to say is that these alternative methods should not be regarded as miracle cure-alls. One of the risks with choosing these alternatives before going to the doctor is that you may not get the correct diagnosis, since the person making the diagnosis in most cases lacks proper medical education. If so, you may not get the proper treatment at the proper time, which may lead to the disease or symptoms getting worse. With this book, I want to present a number of the alternative treatment methods from an evidence-based healthcare point of view. In the conclusion, I will address the idea of possibly integrating some of these alternative methods into the official healthcare system in order to ensure that proper care is given.

Throughout the book, I will present the different methods and describe how they are said to work, what effects they proposedly have and what modern evidence-based research has to say about them. I have chosen to divide the methods into five groups:

- Methods based on the idea that we have an energy body as well as a physical body, and that these two need to be balanced;
- Methods based on various forms of *healing*;
- Methods based on ingesting remedies and preparations that are not conventional pharmaceuticals, e.g. health food and herbal remedies;
- Methods based on stimulating the senses; and
- Methods based on physical activity.

This is an arbitrary division that I have chosen only to make it easier to get an overview. For a lot of the methods, their underlying theories or the way they are practised would make them fit into more than one category. I have also chosen to not rank the methods or categories depending on how effective they seem to be. However, I would like to point out that there are differences between the methods in terms of their effectiveness, as some have a proved positive effect on some ailments, while others probably have no therapeutic effect whatsoever. Moreover, many of the studies that have been conducted are too small or of too poor a quality for researchers to be able to draw any conclusions that can lead to patient recommendations. Some of the methods might even be harmful; there are, for example, preparations among the herbal remedies that are still being marketed, despite evidence of their detrimental effect on health. As a physician, and as a representative of the official healthcare system of Sweden, I can only say that it is up to you if you want to try any of the methods, but that you should always turn to your healthcare team for advice.

Before we move on, I would also like to clarify my position regarding certain terms. So far, I have called the treatment methods I will deal with in this book *alternative methods*. I have done so because that is what they are usually called. Another common term is *alternative medicine*. Using such terms means that you regard these treatments as *alternatives to conventional healthcare and medicines*. I maintain that this is wrong, and that medicine is a profession that involves preventing, diagnosing, and treating diseases and physical injuries. This profession is practised by people with solid education, following extensive ethical rules, and working in regulated institutions. There is no alternative to this. That is why I think the term alternative medicine is wrong. Another term for the methods I will describe in this book is *complementary medicine*, and that is the one I will use for the remainder of the book. I believe that this term better agrees with the use of the methods, since I see them as potential *complements to conventional healthcare and medicines*—at least those methods where research has shown some degree of patient gain, even if it is only "perceived improvement." It is also on this basis that I believe some of the complementary methods could be integrated into the official healthcare system. Some of the methods could be a good complement to the treatments of the official healthcare system, provided that the correct diagnosis is made, that the correct course of treatment is decided upon by medically educated personnel and that the patients themselves ask for these methods as "complements."

I chose the title for the book, *In the Frontier*, because it is my opinion that the research now being done on some of the complementary medical methods is pioneering—in the frontier—in medical science. But my personal desire that the methods that have been proved effective against some ailments should be integrated into the official healthcare system is probably also regarded as push-ing the boundaries of today's Western medical paradigm. In the future, that desire might be more common.

	Evidence-based pharmaceuticals	Tradition-based remedies
Origin	From progressively more accurate planned reviews of earlier plant-based remedies, other research results.	Mainly from very old unplanned tests, on a historical-cultural basis.
Basic purpose	Affect cellular processes with a well-expected positive result for disease control.	Regain the balance in "energetic processes" that have been upset and which hopefully is the basis of diseases.
Effectiveness	Confirmed, both in laboratories and clinically, according to accepted methodology.	Sometimes confirmed in laboratories, but rarely clinically, according to accepted methodology.
Safety	Prescribed by well-educated personnel after a thorough diagnosis of the disease process, based on medical research results.	Prescribed by people who are sometimes skilled in the treatment itself, but who might not understand the fundamental mechanisms of the disease or potential consequences of delayed care.
Research development	Continuous both in terms of improving its resources and the quality/effectiveness of the research methods.	Of lower quality. High enthusiasm but inferior method development.
Research financing	Large grants mainly tied to marketing interests of new products and their introduction in practice.	Much more difficult to receive grants. Research grants mainly come from altruistic financiers.
Health economics	Mostly financed by society, and its activity is completely regulated in terms of social control of costs/marketing results.	Rarely financed by society. "Black market rules" regulate on a significantly higher level.
Attitude of consumers in the West	Most people use these methods/ pharmaceuticals. Distrust is growing.	A smaller number of people use these methods/remedies. The popularity of their benefits grows rapidly but in an unfounded way.

1 Evidence-Based Healthcare or Long Experience?

When you go to the doctor, you can be sure that all the physicians and nurses you meet have a solid education. Every professional in the healthcare sector who has finished their training also receives a permit issued by the authorities to certify that he or she has graduated and completed his or her residency. Furthermore, a check is made against the police record and an individual assessment is made for each applicant. In other words, you can be sure that the people who examine and treat you follow strict regulations and work for your wellbeing. Any pharmaceuticals your doctor prescribes correspond to the diagnosis you have received, and they have a proven effect on the particular condition you suffer from (although they may also affect more parts of your body). All this characterises a scientific and evidence-based healthcare system.

Should you instead go to a therapist working with any of the complementary medical methods, there is no guarantee that the person has a suitable education allowing them to diagnose or treat diseases, physical injuries, or symptoms. Depending on the method, the treatments promise varying degrees of relief or cure. In many cases, too much is promised, which may lead to your not receiving the proper care at the proper time. If you have a serious condition, this could be very dangerous. However, some complementary medical treatments, such as yoga, qigong, acupuncture, and meditation, have proved effective against several ailments and can therefore be recommended by official healthcare providers. For example, acupuncture is today offered by authorised physiotherapists and naprapaths.

Aside from the differences in the healthcare providers' documented competence, there are other fundamental differences between evidence-based healthcare and complementary medicine. One of the most important is the perspective on the processes of disease and recovery. Most complementary medical methods share a basic idea that each individual must come to terms with themselves, achieve personal growth and find balance in life by harmonising opposites. This is the way to recovery, self-healing, and wellbeing. Thus, the key to good health is to be found within ourselves. In contrast, evidence-based medicine regards the process of disease as a result of an aggression from the outside (bacteria, viruses, injuries, accidents etc.) that must be fought by opposites: antihypertensives against hypertension, antibiotics against bacteria, and so on. These opposites battle each other to halt the disease process and ease symptoms, while the sick person is turned into a *patient* (the word comes from Greek and means 'enduring' or 'passive'). The key to good health has been taken from us. Problems are viewed as coming from the outside, and the solution should also come from outside ourselves.

Another fundamental difference between evidence-based healthcare and complementary medicine has to do with the requirements for proof. Most of the complementary methods are based on traditional praxis; that is, a certain method must have been used in the same way for a long time. Usually, it is 30 years in a specific geographical area, but many of the methods, such as yoga and acupuncture, are several thousand years old. Naturally, these may, like everything else, be influenced by the passing of time and the development of ideas in other areas. For example, today we have laser acupuncture, which is a method where an invention in physics is applied to the ancient principles of acupuncture. We can say that complementary medicine is *experience-based*, which means that scientific proof is not a requirement. As opposed to this, evidence-based healthcare is grounded on scientific study results and proof. In order for a result from a study to be regarded as proof, you must be able to perform several studies in the same way and get the same result every time. Such a study is *reproducible*. If you get the same result enough times (and the number differs depending on what you study), the result counts as proof.

This is, of course, a simplified explanation of science, but it is enough to highlight the interesting difference between science and experience. While Western researchers doubt methods that have been used for millennia, they can accept study results which are only 20 years old, as long as they have been sufficiently "proved" through enough studies. I am not saying that this is wrong; on the contrary, evidence-based healthcare is a good and secure system. But I ask you to contemplate whether or not everything really has to be measurable and reproducible. If you think of the different "truths" that have arisen in astronomy over the last few centuries, you probably see my point. When we did not have instruments to look out into space and measure distances, we believed the universe was built in a certain way. But as time passed and our inventions allowed us to learn more and more, our picture of the universe changed, and new "truths" were constantly discovered. So, what about complementary medicine? Would it not be strange if, for example, the Tibetan rites (which I describe in detail later) had no effect whatsoever? If that were the case, why have they survived for millennia, and why are they still practised today? Could it perhaps be that their effectiveness is based on something that our scientists have not yet been able to measure? Or could it be that the effect is achieved over a longer term than the conventional clinical trials extend?

The Tibetan rites, like many of the other Eastern teachings of medicine and exercise, are based on the belief that we humans consist of more than our physical body. We also have a form of life energy. In traditional Chinese medicine, this energy is known as *qi* (pronounced "chi"). In Indian/Tibetan yoga and Ayurveda, it is known as *prana*. Sometimes, it is equalled to what we in the West call a soul or spirit. This energy is said to flow through our body along specific paths, usually called *meridians*, and diseases manifest when the energy flow is blocked for some reason. The goal in many of the Eastern philosophies is that we achieve a balance between our physical body and our energy body, and that the energy is allowed to flow freely along the meridians. When we find this balance and harmony, our body can heal most ailments by itself. Researchers have not been able to measure the qi energy, but that is not to say that it does not exist. What do you think?

When researchers cannot prove the effectiveness of a treatment method through studies, they often claim that the effects are due to *placebo*. In the next chapter, I will explain this concept and ask the question as to whether humans can be taught to heal themselves.

Placebo Effect and Conditioned Self-Healing

A placebo is a preparation or a treatment method without any active substance or therapeutic effect. Placebos are used as a comparative substance when researching the effects of pharmaceuticals. When a patient expects a treatment to have a positive effect, and such an effect occurs even though the treatment does not contain any active substance or therapeutic effect, it is called placebo effect.

The placebo effect might explain patients' perceived improvement after taking sugar pills or having had contact with a charismatic therapist in a grandiose hospital environment.

Between 20 and 40 percent of the effects of various healthcare interventions might be due to placebo effect.

Nocebo is the opposite of placebo, i.e. that negative expectations might lead to negative effects. Incorrect negative information about a disease process may, for example, aggravate symptoms and worsen the patient's perception of the possibility to recover.

2 Placebo Effect
and Conditioned Self-Healing

The word placebo comes from Latin and means "I shall please," or "I shall do good." A placebo is a preparation or a treatment that does not contain any active substances or therapeutic effects. In medical research and the pharmaceutical industry, placebos are used as control substances in drug testing. The placebo can be made to look like the actual drug, and it is then possible to study the differences in effect in the group that receives the drug and the group that only gets the placebo. In this way, the researchers can see just how effective the drug really is. This is what people mean when they talk about "sugar pills"—pills that are made to look like drugs but do not contain any active substances.

In most cases, people who receive sugar pills are not told that it is not the active drug they get. You see, the idea with a placebo is that the one who gets it believes it works. The anticipation that the pill or treatment will work can actually make you experience an improvement, even though no active effect has actually occurred. This is known as the placebo effect. Many researchers claim that the perceived effects from most complementary medical treatments are due to the placebo effect. But the interesting thing is that the placebo effect can be so strong that it actually helps patients get better. Several clinical studies have shown that patients treated only with a placebo experience a significant relief in symptoms. But if it is possible to relieve symptoms through a placebo, which in most cases has no negative side effects, would that not be better than stuffing ourselves with chemical products, the effects of which have not been thoroughly mapped? Some researchers seem to think so, because there are several ongoing studies on the placebo effect.

The first documented use of a placebo in a clinical trial dates to 1801, when British physician John Haygarth showed that a placebo relieved pain just as well as one of the most popular pain treatments of the day, Perkin's metallic tractors. These tractors were rods made of steel, brass and other metal alloys and they were said to "cure pain by extracting the harmful electric fluid that was at the base of all discomfort." Haygarth manufactured wooden rods that were equally effective, thus proving that the positive effects were not due to the healing powers of the metal rods but instead came from the patients' anticipation, hope, and belief that the treatment was effective. Other studies have shown that the relationship between doctor and patient is very important for the recovery process. If a patient goes to a doctor who radiates confidence and security, he or she will recover more quickly than with a doctor who is doubting and insecure. In fact, all of medical history has been characterised by similar studies and fascinating examples of the placebo effect. Some even go as far as to claim that all medical therapy before the 20th century was basically a placebo. Studies conducted during the 1950s estimated that around 40 percent of prescribed drugs were no more effective than placebos. Today, both the manufacturing process and the requirements for the drugs' effectiveness are stricter. But, as I mentioned earlier, it is not as important to map out the drugs' additional effects. You may also wonder why we do not use the placebo effect more often to treat those ailments where it has proved to be effective—even more effective than the drugs that are designed to treat the same ailments. Could it have something to do with economic interests? What do you think?

It is, however, positive to see that today's research on the placebo effect is getting more and more attention. New study results indicate that different forms of placebo treatments could have a significant influence on pain, anxiety, depression, and substance abuse. There are also studies showing that sham surgery (surgery where the actual therapeutically effective step is omitted) could be effective. In one case, a man with Parkinson's disease had a sham surgery, and his symptoms showed a significant improvement. Another study has shown that sham surgery of knees with mock knee washouts are just as effective as real procedures. In addition, positive effects have been observed on various biological systems such as the respiratory organs, immune system and endocrine system. According to some studies, as much as 20 to 40 percent of the effects of modern pharmaceuticals may be due to placebo, despite a proven active substance in the drugs.

There are, of course, opponents, and they claim that the positive results observed from placebo in reality are a combination of the patients' spontaneous improvement, positive results from other treatments given at the same time and other causes. They contend that only a fraction of the positive results is due to placebo effect, and then only in the treatment of subjective parameters such as pain. However, some studies have shown that the effects from placebo are actually clearest when assessing physical and measurable parameters, such as blood pressure and asthma.

The opposite of the placebo effect is called nocebo effect, and it means that our condition can actually deteriorate if we are convinced that things will go badly. There are some cases where it is believed that a wrong diagnosis led to a worse condition because the patient expected to get worse, or had even given up hope after receiving the negative information. Since ethical reasons make it more difficult to study the nocebo effect, we do not know as much about it. But we do know that the part in our brain that is related to memories and anxiety can make pain worse.

Can We Heal Ourselves?

Expectations can release hormonal changes and biochemical reactions, which alter the bodily functions. After a while, a learning system can be built up, which starts a chain reaction from simpler signals—a so-called conditioning process. This has been proven to change immune responses and can even be set off and enhanced by social pressure, both positively and negatively.

In other words, it seems as if the body can be trained to heal itself by expecting healing. This raises a number of intriguing questions for the future.

Can We Heal Ourselves?

So, what happens in us when we "only think" that a treatment or a substance benefits us? In one study, where X-rays were taken of the participants' brains, it showed that they produced opioids, an analgesic hormone, and released them when they expected an analgesic effect from a preparation that was actually placebo. Other so-called neuromodulators were also released, such as cholecystokinin, cannabinoids, and dopamine. Several studies have shown that the release of these neuromodulators in turn lead to important changes in the central nervous system, for example in the prefrontal cortex in the brain, in the limbic system, and in thalamus. Other so-called subcortical systems are also affected, such as hypothalamus and the amygdala. So, what does all this mean? Well, it means that it seems like we medicate ourselves when we expect pain relief. It is not only that we think we get better; this belief seems to activate biochemical reactions in us that actually make us better.

If the expectations are fulfilled, the placebo effect is further strengthened through a kind of associative learning, which researchers call *Pavlovian conditioning*. The term comes from a classic experiment in psychology where the Russian Nobel Prize winner Ivan Pavlov made his dogs drool simply by ringing a bell. At first, the dogs drooled when they saw food. What Pavlov did was to ring the bell before feeding the dogs. After a while, the dogs learned to associate the sound of the bell with food, and in the end, it was enough to ring the bell: the dogs would drool without any food present. Such learning, or conditioning, can happen in many areas, and researchers now claim that the placebo effect can be enhanced through it.

Several recent experiments have shown that the immune system can be improved through conditioning. Both humans and animals can learn to change their immune response when given an inactive substance that was previously associated with a suppressor or an enhancer of the immune response. In other words, the immune system can learn from experience and respond in an almost reflective manner, just like Pavlov's dogs learned to drool at the sound of the bell. The immune response is thus related to behaviour, and these discoveries have given rise to a whole new field in medicine, known as psychoneuroimmunology.

In recent years, it has been observed that patients can experience placebo effects only by noticing a positive effect in another person undergoing analgesic treatment. Thus, it might be possible that the information needed to build up expectations of pain relief can be received through *social learning*. In fact, studies have shown that peer pressure enhances the placebo effect. For example, for religious people who are surrounded by others holding the same beliefs, the strength of the placebo effect from healing treatments and experiences is increased. However, healing based on faith needs both a good "story" and an active listener; that is, the person about to be healed needs to believe in the healing message.

You could say that the person treated with placebo responds to the form of the treatment and not to the content, since the content is ineffective. This means that external factors, such as the place of the treatment and the relationship between the therapist and the treated person, are of great significance. As I mentioned earlier, other studies have shown that the relationship between doctor and patient is important, and so is, for example, the relationship between a spiritual leader/healer and a believer. It even seems as if a trustful and supportive relationship between therapist and treated is the most important factor for the placebo effect to work. Recent studies indicate that placebo can work even when the participants *know that they are receiving a placebo treatment*. A positive effect from the treatment could still be observed, but it was believed to be due to the well-established relationship between the therapist and the participants.

What, then, can be the practical use of all this? It is impossible to answer that until we have more information. But the results from the studies mentioned above raise a whole lot of questions. How much more effort should we put into building good relationships between therapists and people receiving treatment? If a patient's faith in a treatment or substance can realise an expected effect, can this be used for therapeutic purposes on a more general level? And if placebo is enough to relieve symptoms, does it really matter whether the proposed effectiveness of the complementary medical treatments is based on energies we cannot measure or on placebo? Perhaps the most intriguing question of all is about what we may call *conditioned self-healing*: if it is correct to assume that the placebo effect can be used to effectively treat various organ systems, can people then be conditioned to treat or cure their diseases and ailments without pharmaceutical preparations? In other words, can people be taught to heal themselves? It remains to be seen, and we live in a very exciting age when Western science and Eastern experience are moving towards a union.

Balancing the Physical Body and Life Energy

The most important and statistically most common methods used in complementary medicine are based on a dualistic perspective on life and the human body—except for our physical body, we also consist of an energy body. Good health is achieved when these two are balanced, and diseases occur because of imbalances or disruptions in the energy. This life energy goes under different names within different traditions, but it is somewhat comparable to what we in the West call soul or spirit.

3 Balancing the Physical Body and Life Energy

As I mentioned in Chapter 1, many of the complementary medical treatments are based on the idea that our bodies consist of more than our physical form, that we also have a spirit, soul, or life energy. In this chapter, I have gathered methods that are based on this belief. Most of them have a long tradition in Asia, primarily through traditional Chinese medicine and Indian-Tibetan teachings of yoga and Ayurveda (traditional Indian medicine). They are in different ways connected to the Eastern philosophies/religions known as Hinduism, Buddhism, Taoism, and Confucianism. I will not describe these religious-philosophical systems in detail, as thorough descriptions of them can be found elsewhere. But I will mention that traditional Chinese medicine is primarily based on Taoist and Confucianist ideas, whereas yoga is linked to Buddhist and Hindu teachings.

Traditional Chinese medicine is based on 2,500 years of experience in herbal medicine, massage, acupuncture, and movement therapies such as qigong. It is also influenced by modern clinical research. One of the most important fundamental ideas is the theory of the qi energy flowing through meridians in our bodies and permeating all living things. It links us to the rest of the universe, to our fellow humans, and all other creatures. Another important principle is the balance between the two universal forces known as *yin* and *yang*. These two opposites are said to give rise to all processes in the universe, and they manifest as more or less tangible dualities, such as light and darkness, or fire and water. I will describe this a little more closely in the section on qigong and tai chi. In traditional Chinese medicine, health is regarded as a state of harmony and balance. Attaining good health is largely about finding the balance between *yin* and *yang*, and harmonising the body's qi energy, allowing it to flow freely.

In the Indian-Tibetan traditions, the life energy is called *prana*. It is a term that encompasses all the cosmic energy, which is said to permeate the universe and all things, both inanimate and animate. This includes the human life force, manifested in the breathing (I describe this in more detail in the section called *Respiratory Training*).

The two terms, qi and prana, are thus rather similar, and they are to a certain degree comparable to what we in the West usually refer to as a soul or spirit. Regardless if you believe in such a life energy or not, it could be worthwhile to try a few of the training methods described in this chapter. Science has not been able to measure or observe any form of life energy, so researchers are doubtful of the theories that form the basis for the Eastern training philosophies. But the purely physical aspects have proved beneficial, so even if you do not agree with the ideas behind yoga, qigong, or acupuncture, their physiological effects might still help you battle certain ailments. However, it is always best to consult your healthcare team prior to trying any complementary medical treatments.

Yoga

In the West, yoga is often regarded as merely a form of exercise, but it is really a complete philosophy of life, which includes approaches aimed at maintaining and promoting good health.

Some researchers claim that meditative movement therapies have a positive effect on cortical and subcortical structures in the brain. When these systems become activated, the level of stress hormones is reduced, and it has a positive effect on the immune system.

Studies indicate that yoga seems to have positive effects on a wide range of ailments and diseases.

Western researchers have not been able to determine a clear mechanism behind the physiological effects of yoga. The most common negative side effects reported include muscle strains and ligament injuries.

Be sure to consult your healthcare team if you wish to begin with yoga and simultaneously use psychotropic medications, or antidepressants.

Yoga

Among the Eastern philosophies, yoga is perhaps the most widespread and practised in the West. Yoga is actually a collective name denoting an entire group of physical, mental, and spiritual disciplines tied to Hindu, Buddhist, and Jain traditions. The word comes from the ancient language known as Sanskrit, which is related to the ancient Indic languages. *Yoga* is derived from the root *yuj*, meaning "to tie, unite, link together." The way you practise yoga can look very differently depending on which discipline you follow, but the overall purpose of yoga is to unite the physical, mental, and spiritual worlds into one cohesive and independent unit, and thus achieve absolute freedom. Aside from this spiritual goal, many people practise yoga to reduce stress, keep the body agile, and increase wellbeing.

Yoga originates in ancient India, and it is one of the six major Hindu philosophical schools. Like the other schools, yoga is largely based on the four Vedic scriptures known as the Vedas. They are ancient religious texts written in Sanskrit and their teachings are still practised today. There are also similarities between the Vedic priests' meditative and physical exercises and many of the practical exercises in yoga. All of the six Hindu schools of philosophy emphasise the importance of tolerance and respect for different perspectives and religious beliefs. Another common denominator is the belief in a cyclical world with reincarnation (rebirth) in various forms. Other important concepts in yoga include balance, harmony and moderation. These are concepts that appeal to a lot of people, and perhaps this is one of the reasons why yoga has become so popular in the West.

The oldest of the Vedas date to roughly 1700 to 1100 BCE, but yoga seems to be older than that. Archaeological discoveries in the form of seals, dated to around 2500 BCE, show figures in what appears to be yogic postures. However, the first written source to specifically mention yoga is the *Upanishads*, the oldest part of which dates to the 6th century BCE. A couple of centuries later, a more complete and systematic description was written down, and it can be found in Patanjali's *Yoga Sutras*. This text has not been precisely dated, but researchers claim that it was written sometime between the 3rd century BCE and the 6th century CE. Early Buddhist texts contain similar systematic descriptions of yoga, for example the *P li Canon*, written down in 29 BCE. Historically, yoga is said to be comprised of eight components, which Patanjali describes in his *Yoga Sutras*. He states that the eight components are:

- Moral discipline (yama);
- Self-study, purity and virtuous habits (niyama);
- Physical exercises/postures (asana);
- Breath control (pranayama);
- Withdrawal from sensory impressions (pratyahara);
- Concentration (dharana);
- Meditation (dhyana); and
- Happiness/peace of mind (samadhi).

Yoga is still most widespread in India, Nepal, and large parts of Southeast Asia. But thanks to key figures like Swami Vivekananda and other Hindu monks who migrated and brought yoga to the West, the various yogic disciplines have become internationally known.

Hatha yoga, which is a combination of asana and pranayama, i.e. various physical exercises and breathing techniques, is the most well-known form of yoga in the West. In recent years, some adapted forms of yoga have become popular. One example of this is the so-called *office yoga*, a kind of yoga that can be practised while you are at your office, even while you remain seated on your work chair. If you have a sedentary job, this could be a good way to integrate a little physical activity into your workday. Office yoga often consists of exercises from the *kundalini* style of yoga, which is a combination of light movement, meditation, and breathing techniques.

Practising yoga is rarely associated with negative side effects, but remember that, like with any other physical activity, it is not without risk. The most commonly reported adverse effects are muscle strains and ligament injuries. In view of the large number of practitioners around the world, relatively few serious adverse effects are reported, and most of these occur because people show reckless behaviour or neglect their basic medical condition. Be sure to consult your healthcare team if you want to begin practising yoga and are currently using psychotropic medications, e.g. antidepressants. If you want to try yoga, you should also make sure to contact a qualified instructor, and as a beginner, you should avoid advanced exercises such as headstand, lotus position, and intense breathing techniques. As your body becomes more agile and you gain experience, you may move on to more advanced yoga techniques.

Evidence-based research finds it difficult to study the health benefits from yoga because it contains so many different therapies which are often given at the same time. Yoga is also used as a complement to conventional pharmaceuticals, which makes it difficult to distinguish the positive effects and put them in relation with the different treatments. In other words, it is difficult to tell which positive effect comes from which exercise in yoga, or, in cases where the two are combined, if the effect primarily comes from the drugs.

Researchers have not been able to explain the physiological mechanisms behind the effects of yoga. Without going into too much detail, I can say that different researchers have set forth several different explanations, but none of them can singlehandedly clarify the effects that yoga seems to have. Some researchers claim that all of the so-called meditative movement therapies (yoga, qigong, tai chi etc.) have a positive influence on the cortical and sub-cortical structures in the brain. When these systems activate, the number of stress hormones are reduced, and the immune system also benefits. These therapies are also regarded as influencing the nervous system in a way that promotes physical wellbeing.

In recent years, a lot of effort has been put into researching yoga, and the results indicate that it might have positive effects as a complement in the treatment of carpal tunnel syndrome, fibromyalgia, and chronic back pain. The quality of life seems to increase for fatigued cancer patients who begin to practise yoga. The same goes for the elderly, where researchers have seen positive effects on physical function, mental health, and quality of sleep. Other studies suggest that yoga seems to have a positive effect on several different ailments, such as stress, depression, eating disorders, labour pain, osteoarthritis, chronic kidney disease, hypertension, diabetes, and epilepsy. Yoga also seems to be a good complement in the rehabilitation of stroke patients, where the study results indicate improved cognition, mood, and balance, as well as reduced stress. New studies are published daily, and I look forward to the new results. However, it is important to remember that most studies so far have been of poor quality, and the healthcare system cannot therefore give any general recommendations. But considering that this ancient and virtually side effect-free method is practised by close to 300 million people worldwide, it should not be long until it can be integrated into the official healthcare system.

Vyayam

Vyayam is similar to yoga, tai chi, and qigong, but so far, there are no studies on this particular method and its potential effects on health.

Vyayam

Vyayam is a dynamic form of yoga with elements from Indian dancing, traditional Ayurvedic medicine, and mysticism from the tantric yoga. The word is a Sanskrit compound consisting of *vyu* (meaning "pushing the air" or "guiding the breath") and *yama* (meaning "control"). Practitioners claim that vyayam is about taming the energy that comes to us via the air through our breathing.

Vyayam is a collection of breathing techniques, body movements, and meditation. The purpose of the exercises is to bring about a state of mind that enhances our inner balance, reduces stress, has a liberating effect, maximizes the feeling of creativity and spontaneity, and makes the muscles more elastic and the joints more flexible. All of this supposedly leads to reduced pain and an increased overall wellbeing. A crucial element is the idea that you can control your consciousness by controlling your breathing. It is this breath control that, together with precise body movements and meditation, will create an intimate connection between the body, the consciousness, and the energy.

Vyayam has a lot in common with yoga, tai chi, and qigong, but as of yet, no studies have been conducted on vyayam and its potential health benefits. As with yoga, if you are interested in trying vyayam, you should find a qualified instructor to guide you. You should also consult your healthcare team about this form of exercise, especially if you are currently using any psychotropic medications or are pregnant.

> **Tibetan Rites**
>
> The Tibetan rites are based on the belief that the human body contains seven wheels that always spin and keep us healthy. As we become older, these wheels spin slower. The rites are supposed to counteract this and thus keep us young and strong. The rites are similar to yoga even though their origins are debated.
>
> The Tibetan rites include spinning and sometimes intense exercises, so you should be careful if you want to try them.
>
> As of today, there are no scientific evidence of the rites' effects.

Tibetan Rites

The Tibetan rites were described for the first time in 1939 in the book *The Eye of Revelation* by American Peter Kelder. In the book, he claimed that he had encountered a retired British army officer who had been stationed in India. This officer, called Colonel Bradford (probably a pseudonym), had heard stories of a group of Tibetan monks who had discovered a kind of "fountain of youth". The stories told of elderly people who became healthy, strong, and full of vitality after having visited a certain monastery. Bradford then went up into the Himalayas in search of the monks, and he eventually found them. He saw that they appeared very healthy and younger than their actual age. The monks' secret proved to be a special sequence of yoga exercises that was said to be more than 2,000 years old. Colonel Bradford learned the technique and practiced the rites daily for five minutes. After some time, he decided to reunite with his Western lifestyle and dedicate his life to spreading the knowledge of the five rites.

There is no telling whether the story in Kelder's book is true or not, and it is also uncertain how the Tibetan rites came to be, but they are very similar to certain exercises from the traditional Tibetan yoga. The difference between Indian and Tibetan yoga is that the latter is based on a flowing sequence of motions while Indian yoga is often based on static positions. However, certain sources claim that the Tibetan rites predate yoga with more than 700 years, and that their origin can instead be found in *Kum Nye*, which are ancient Tibetan medicinal-religious exercises. We may never know the truth, and when questioned, Tibetan lamas say only that the origins of the rites are not important; what is important is the effect you get from only practicing them for five to 10 minutes daily.

The Tibetan rites are based on the belief that there are seven wheels in the human body that constantly spin. As we grow older, the wheels spin more slowly. The rites will counteract this and keep us young and strong. They are said to purify the skin and make the hair fuller. They soften up joints and muscles, reduce fat deposits in the hypodermis, improve certain sensory functions, and balance mental processes. As of today, there is no evidence-based research on the proposed beneficial effects of the rites. The five rites are as follows:

> **First Rite**: a spinning exercise where you hold out your arms horizontally and spin in a clockwise direction (from left to right) until you become slightly dizzy. This exercise is supposed to make the wheels in the body spin faster.

> **Second Rite**: similar to regular leg lifts, you lie on your back with your arms outstretched along your body. Lift your legs until they point upwards at a 90-degree angle to your body. If you are able, it is good to push a little farther. Keep your legs in this position for a few seconds before you slowly lower them again. Let all muscles relax and then repeat. It is also good to raise your head while you lift your legs, and lower it as you lower your legs.

> **Third Rite**: kneel and keep your arms vertical against the side of your legs. Move your hands to your lower back and

bend backwards from the waist as much as you are able (you can use your toes for support). Also bend your neck as far back as possible. When you straighten up, let your arms return to the vertical position. Bend your neck slightly forward until your chin touches your chest. Resume the straight-up position and relax for a few seconds before you repeat the exercise. The idea behind this rite is to draw energy in through the navel, which according to certain philosophers is the very part of the body where life begins.

Fourth Rite: sit with your legs outstretched before you and your hands on the floor. Keep your fingers together and angle them slightly away from your body. It is important that the legs are absolutely straight, with the back of the legs as close to the floor as possible. Rest your chin against your chest. Now push your body up as far as possible, rising on toes and hands, until you reach a bridge pose. Your knees should be bent so that your legs form a 90-degree angle. Bend your head back as far as possible when the body is in this position. Maintain the position for a few seconds before you resume the sitting position. Let your body relax before you repeat the exercise. This rite is supposed to create a flow of energy from the loins down through the legs.

Fifth Rite: begin from a position similar to a push-up, with your feet about 30 cm apart. Instead of going down, as in a push-up, raise your butt in the air until your body draws an up-side-down V. Then lower your body without touching the floor and push your head forwards. This creates a swinging motion that is believed to quicken the spinning of the wheels.

The Tibetan rites are similar to yoga, and the effects that practitioners claim to feel are often the same as for yoga, tai chi and qigong. But so far, no research has been done on the health effects of the Tibetan rites, and therefore the healthcare system cannot recommend them as complementary treatment. As with yoga, tai chi, and qigong, the risk of side effects is not that great, but since the Tibetan rites contain spinning and sometimes intense exercises, you should use caution if you decide to try them. You should consult your healthcare team if you are interested in these exercises while you are pregnant, and you should avoid them if you are currently using psychotropic medications.

Qigong and Tai Chi

Both qigong and tai chi combine movement, postures, breathing exercises and meditation.

Research has shown positive results in elderly people with balance problems, and also on rheumatic ailments, chronic fatigue, dementia, depression, and COPD. Studies indicate that qigong and tai chi can enhance the immune system. Tai chi also seems to be an effective complementary therapy for people with Parkinson's disease. Several studies have shown that practising tai chi gives better motor function and balance.

It has not been determined whether the effects are due to the physical activity, relaxation, balancing of energy, or placebo.

Qigong and Tai Chi

If you have ever been to China and gone out in the early morning, you have probably seen groups of people—often elderly—practising qigong. It is a training philosophy that belongs to the traditional Chinese medicine. The word qigong can be spelled differently depending on how you transliterate the Chinese characters into our Latin alphabet, but I have chosen this spelling because it is probably the most common. The meaning of the word is something like "cultivating the life energy" (*qi*, as you remember, is the life energy), and the purpose of the training is to balance the body's energy through a combination of movement, postures, breathing, and meditation. Advocates of qigong claim that the practice leads to balance and harmony between body and mind, and that it benefits the body's own physiological and psychological mechanisms for self-healing. As in the yogic philosophy, it is believed that health is a state of dynamic balance, and that the training helps in preventing imbalances that manifest as diseases and other ailments.

According to historians, qigong may be as old as 7,000 years. The oldest archaeological find portraying qigong is an urn of that age that was discovered in northern China in 1982. It is believed that similar exercises were practised by shamanistic priests in order to reach a state of trance. The oldest written source that describes qigong is the book *Huangdi Neijing*, which is around 2,000 years old. In English, the book is usually called "The Yellow Emperor's Classic of Internal Medicine." In Chinese mythology, the Yellow Emperor is one of the mythological rulers of ancient China. The book is one of the cornerstones of traditional Chinese medicine and a much-read text, even today. Other texts, such as the works of philosophers, like Confucius, Lao Tzu, and Chuang Tzu, have also shaped the qigong that we see today.

Tai chi is a similar form of training, but it is at its core a martial art where physical and mental training are practised in ways similar to qigong. Tai chi is actually a short form for *tai chi chuan* (pronounced "tie jee chuann"), and it is difficult to offer a simple translation of the meaning. If you look up the term on the Internet, you will find many sources claiming that it means something like "the ultimate boxing" or "the ultimate fist." But that is only partly true. Tai chi is a term from the Taoist philosophy. Taoism is an ancient naturalistic and spiritual Chinese philosophy. Taoists believe that before the universe came into existence, the cosmos existed in a state of *wu chi* or nothingness (*wu chi* literally means "no polarity"). Then a change occurred, and the cosmos became divided into two parts, *wu chi* and the changed part known as *tai chi* (literally "great polarity). The opposite poles of this changed part are known as *yin* and *yang*, and they are the two fundamental opposites that give rise to all processes in the universe. Thus, you should not confuse *chi* with the life energy *qi*. They are two completely different words in Chinese! However, the idea that the qi energy permeates everything, including our bodies, is prevalent in tai chi as well.

So, what does *chuan* mean? Literally, it means "fist," but it is a word that implies that something has to do with martial arts. For example, there is another form of martial arts (a style of kung fu) known as *bai he chuan*, where *bai he* means "white crane" and the whole compound means the style of fighting that is inspired by the crane's movements and nature. Thus, *tai chi chuan* is the martial art in the state of change from no polarity to great polarity. This may sound complicated, but the main concept centres around a change in the balance between *yin* and *yang*. The aim is to understand this balance in yourself in order to create a change when needed. When tai chi is practised as a martial art, you extend this change to influence your opponent's balance. But the idea is that you can also use tai chi to affect the balance between *yin* and *yang* in anything outside yourself, such as your lifestyle, work and opportunities in life.

Qigong and tai chi both share a close connection with Taoism, but also with Confucianism, which is another ancient Chinese philosophy. Both of these philosophies emphasise the importance of the natural laws and encourage us to work with nature and its laws instead of resisting them. The human body is viewed as a microscopic mirror reflection of the universe, and the energy that permeates our bodies also links us to the whole universe. Thus, it is not only for our own sake that we should find a balance; in the long term, it also benefits other people, as well as nature and the whole world.

The number of qigong and tai chi practitioners around the world is very large— approximately 250 million people according to some sources. Most practitioners are found in China and East Asia, where qigong and tai chi are among the most common forms of regular exercise.

In recent years, Western researchers have shown an increased interest in studying the health benefits of qigong and tai chi. So far, the research has shown positive results for elderly people with balance problems. Positive results have also been seen for rheumatic problems, chronic fatigue, dementia, depression, and chronic obstructive pulmonary disease. There are also studies indicating that qigong and tai chi might enhance the immune system. Tai chi also seems to be an effective complementary treatment for people with Parkinson's disease, since a number of studies have shown that the practice leads to better motor functions and balance.

However, researchers say that it is difficult to pinpoint what it is that gives the positive effects. Both qigong and tai chi combine movement, meditation and a belief in the qi energy and its importance for our health. Also, researchers have not been able to measure and quantify the qi energy, and therefore they cannot explain the mechanisms behind the effects. This means that it is difficult to determine whether the effects come from physical activity, relaxation, balancing the body's energy or from placebo. Or perhaps it is the combination? No matter where the effects come from, qigong is an accepted form of physical activity in the Swedish healthcare system, and Swedes can get qigong as physical activity on prescription (PAP). Perhaps more countries will implement this in the near future? If you want to try qigong, make sure to contact a qualified instructor, and consult your healthcare team if you are pregnant.

Respiratory Training

Respiratory training seems to improve lung function in patients with MS and Parkinson's disease, help patients with heart failure, patients who have suffered a stroke, or offer a good complement in the treatment of COPD and various forms of cancer.

Reports show that completely healthy individuals also benefit from respiratory training. However, the studies conducted so far do not meet the strict requirements set up by evidence-based healthcare. Therefore, no recommendations for respiratory training can be given until more research has been conducted.

Few studies report any side effects from respiratory training.

Respiratory Training

In complementary medicine, respiratory training is a collective name denoting a number of different breathing techniques that mostly originate in yogic traditions. In yoga, such respiratory training is known as *pranayama*, which is a word that does not translate easily. It is often said to mean "breath control," but that does not quite cover it. The word is a compound, with one part being *prana*, which means "life force," especially in the form of breathing, but, in a wider sense, all cosmic energy. The other part is either *yama*, meaning "control" or *ayama*, which means "expansion." Pranayama thus means that you control and/or expand your life energy by controlling your breathing in various ways.

This respiratory training can trace its origins to Buddhism, and a number of different techniques are described in texts that are more than 2,500 years old. Some sources describe respiratory training as a method of its own—a method for reducing stress, increasing concentration, and finding an inner calm. Other sources regard the training as a part of other, more extensive training methods, such as yoga and tai chi. In recent years, respiratory training has also featured as a part of mindfulness, and physiotherapists use respiratory training techniques in the treatment of chronic pulmonary disease.

The purpose of respiratory training in complementary medicine is to regain the body's energy balance through controlled breathing, primarily by regulating stress levels in order to treat physical ailments. Breathing is regarded as the most immediate of all vital functions and to practise controlled breathing is said to have several positive effects. Among other things, it is said to:

- Help you relax;
- Be a tool for training your abdominal and respiratory muscles;
- Reduce stress;
- Help you lose weight;
- Improve lung function;
- Stabilise blood pressure;
- Improve muscle performance;
- Improve sleep;
- Improve sex life;
- Relieve pain; and
- Help you feel more energetic and increase your spiritual growth.

Today, there are several different techniques and types of training used for enhancing the respiratory muscles and lung capacity. It is therefore difficult to specify when and how a certain technique should be used to achieve the best possible result. However, recent research has presented a number of interesting reports indicating that techniques such as RMT (Respiratory Muscle Training), NIPPV (Non-Invasive Positive Pressure Ventilation), ACBT (Active Cycle of Breathing Techniques), pranayama, the Buteyko method, and diaphragmatic breathing can be of great use to certain patient groups. But that is not all. These reports also show that completely healthy individuals can benefit from the exercises. However, the studies do not meet the strict requirements that evidence-based research has put up, and therefore, the healthcare system cannot recommend respiratory training until more studies have been conducted. I can, however, mention a few areas where studies indicate positive results. Just remember that these results are very unclear.

One study suggests that the breathing technique known as IMT (inspiratory muscle training) may improve lung function in patients with MS and Parkinson's disease. IMT also seems to be a method that may help patients with heart failure and those who have suffered a stroke. Respiratory training could also be a good complement in the treatment of asthma, cystic fibrosis, and COPD (chronic obstructive pulmonary disease), but it does not seem to have any effect in the treatment of pneumonia. Lastly, there are several studies indicating that respiratory training may be a good complement in the treatment of various cancers, since it seems to increase the patients' quality of life.

Researchers have so far not been able to explain the mechanisms behind the effects of respiratory training, but it is believed that there are many factors involved. Even though we do not know exactly how it happens, it seems respiratory training has a positive effect on the strength of the respiratory muscles, lung capacity and lung function in general. Naturally, improving lung function is a good thing, and since there are very few studies reporting any negative side effects from respiratory training, it may well be a method that could complement more evidence-based treatment methods.

Acupuncture

Like qigong, acupuncture is one of the cornerstones of traditional Chinese
medicine, and it is also described in "The Yellow Emperor's Classic of Internal
Medicine." However, the word we use is derived from the Latin *acus* (needle)
and *punctura* (prick, penetrate). An acupuncture treatment consists of pricking
the skin with needles in specific places, known as acupuncture points. If you
do not like needles, there are other ways of trying acupuncture. The points
can be stimulated with magnets, ultrasound, low power laser, electric current,
or simply with your hands (this last method is described in more detail under
Acupressure). As acupuncture spread from China to Korea, Japan, Vietnam, and

later to France and other Western countries, a number of different "schools" were founded. All of the above countries have their own acupuncture traditions, even France, where they specialise in ear acupuncture. In recent years, acupuncture has meshed with modern technology, giving us such adaptations as laser acupuncture.

No matter which technique you apply, the basic belief in acupuncture is that diseases and other ailments are caused by various imbalances in the body. The qi energy is perhaps blocked from flowing freely along the body's meridians. Or perhaps there is an imbalance between *yin* and *yang*, or an uneven influence from one of the five elements wood, water, fire, earth, and metal. For example, it is said that some diseases are caused by wind, cold, and water having disrupted certain meridians. The aim is then to treat these meridians in a way that restores the balance between the elements. Thus, the purpose of an acupuncture treatment is to restore the balance by stimulating the correct acupuncture point in the correct manner. Good health is equated with good balance and harmony, and if you achieve this, the body will self-heal. The number of acupuncture points on the body is uncertain. According to early sources, there were 365 of them, but over the centuries, more and more have been listed, and today, practitioners speak of more than 2,000 points. These are said to be distributed along 14 meridians, half of which are classed as *yin* and half as *yang*.

Many countries offer acupuncture treatment through authorised healthcare providers, such as physiotherapists and naprapaths. Treatment is then usually given without focussing on the energy balance; instead, Western acupuncture is founded on evidence-based research. The points to be stimulated are chosen depending on the so-called anatomical nerve supply to the organ you want to treat. If, for example, you want to treat the uterus, you choose a point on the body from where nerves reach the uterus. When you activate the nerves and muscles in this way, signals are sent to the spinal cord. The signals in turn activate the brain and various cytokine and hormone systems. So, you could say that the physiological effects of acupuncture have been proven, even if the traditional theories behind the method are still in question. It is interesting that Western medicine bases acupuncture on nerve impulses, which is electrical energy, when Eastern acupuncture likewise speaks of energy flowing through the body. As I mentioned earlier, researchers have not been able to measure the qi energy, but I think it is an interesting coincidence. Thus, we do not yet know if it is only nerve impulses or if there is also an additional form of energy that is stimulated by acupuncture. But the main point is that a lot of people feel that the treatment helps them in relieving pain and disease.

There is ongoing research on acupuncture, and it is one of the most explored methods of complementary medicine. There are tens of thousands of texts on acupuncture from the centuries before modern time, and there are also a great number of modern research studies. One thing that makes it difficult to study acupuncture in general is that there are many different techniques and practices. Over the centuries, practitioners have edited descriptions of methods and added personal interpretations, comments, and clinical experiences. This has led to some confusion, and, for example, one ailment may be described in different ways with different points to be stimulated. This makes it difficult to create a systematic and general description of how acupuncture should be practised.

Despite these difficulties, modern research has been able to prove that acupuncture has positive effects on a number of ailments. Furthermore, acupuncture is regarded as much better than some pharmaceuticals when it comes to negative side effects, and in many cases, it has proved more effective than the placebo treatments it was compared to. Research has found that acupuncture may be effective for:

- A range of so-called musculoskeletal ailments, such as osteoarthritis, neck pain, back pain, sciatica, and whiplash;
- Nausea and vomiting (e.g. in cancer patients and post-operative patients);
- Headache;
- Obesity;
- Constipation, IBS, and IBD (better effect than pharmaceuticals);
- Pain relief (in general, and especially during childbirth and endoscopic examinations);
- Prevention of angina;
- Autism and ADHD;

- Clinical depression (as effective as pharmaceuticals, but without negative side effects);
- Schizophrenia;
- PMS and menstrual pain;
- Erection problems and chronic prostatitis;
- Asthma; and
- Shingles.

However, it is important to point out that many studies suffer from poor design, scale, or methodology, and it is therefore impossible to draw any clear conclusions. But, since there are so few negative side effects from acupuncture and since it has proved a cost-efficient form of treatment, it is not surprising that the Swedish healthcare system has accepted acupuncture. Perhaps the healthcare systems in more countries will follow. The World Health Organization has listed quality requirements that acupuncture educations should meet to guarantee a high standard and basis in the healthcare system. Make sure you contact an authorised healthcare provider if you decide to try acupuncture.

Acupressure

Acupressure is based on the same theories as acupuncture, but instead of needles, pressure is used; thus, it can be regarded as a form of massage.

The World Health Organization has presented a list of 43 areas of use for acupressure and acupuncture. Here, the methods are said to be effective against hay fever, toothache, kidney and gallstones, high and low blood pressure, tennis elbow, depression, and pain in the head, neck, and back.

Acupressure is a safe treatment method.

Acupressure

If you do not feel like getting pricked by needles but still want to try a treatment similar to acupuncture, then acupressure is for you. This treatment method is based on the same theories as acupuncture and is said to have the same effects. The difference is that instead of stimulating the acupuncture point with needles, the practitioner presses with his/her fingers on the points to resolve pain. A similar treatment method is called *trigger point therapy*, which a naprapath may employ. Another similar method is called *energy massage*. It is a form of body massage that activates the acupuncture points in your body, thus increasing your energy.

As with acupuncture, a lot of research is being conducted on acupressure. For example, researchers at Karolinska Institutet in Stockholm, Sweden, are studying the effects of acupressure treatment of women at childbirth. As early as 1979, the World Health Organization presented a list of 43 indications (areas of use) for acupressure and acupuncture, where the areas were given different colours depending on how effective the treatment was considered to be. The areas given a green colour (i.e. where the treatment proved effective) included:

- Hay fever;
- Toothache;
- Kidney and gallstones;
- High and low blood pressure;
- Tennis elbow;
- Pain in the head, neck, and back; and
- Depression.

Acupressure has no actual side effects and is therefore regarded as a safe treatment method. There are a few unusual side effects, including temporary insomnia and headache.

> If you want to read more about acupressure and how you may treat different points on your body, I refer you to my book about acupressure, *Feelless*.

Reflexology

Reflexology is the international name for zone therapy, and the method is based on treating zones on the body which are said to be connected to various organs. A treatment consists of massaging points connected to these zones and organs, since it is believed that these points ache when an ailment affects the related organ. However, a treatment involves the entire zone (not only certain points), and it is pressure massaged up to perceived pain threshold. Thus, a reflexology treatment is different from an acupressure treatment. The underlying theories of reflexology also differ from the theories on which acupressure and acupuncture are based. Research has shown that the effects of reflexology are not nearly as clear as they are with acupressure and acupuncture.

It is said that reflexology can relieve a number of ailments such as various forms of pain, hormonal problems, skin problems, asthma, allergies, sleep disorders, and recurring infections, but in view of the studies conducted so far, it is uncertain whether reflexology is effective or not.

Some studies have even shown negative effects, and therefore, you are recommended to instead try regular massage or acupressure/acupuncture if you suffer from an ailment for which these treatment methods have documented positive effects.

Reflexology

Reflexology is a therapy that is based on the belief that the body can be divided into vertical layers, or zones, from head to feet. Thus, another word for reflexology is zone therapy. Each zone governs the body parts and organs that it encompasses. There are also points on the body, known as reflex points, that are linked to the different zones and organs. If there is an imbalance, strain, or disease affecting a specific part of the body, it manifests as pain in the respective zone and reflex point. The sore point is then massaged with the purpose of increasing the flow of blood and energy to the afflicted area. The idea is that this resolves blockages, clears out toxins and waste products, and activates the body's own natural ability to self-heal. You may also feel a deep relaxation, which is a prerequisite for recovery. The massage can be given either by hand or by using special reflexology tools.

Advocates of reflexology claim that the human body has a well-developed communication network, not only for blood, lymph, and nerves, but also via the energy meridians. The zones on the body are thus said to communicate through energy with glands, organs and all parts of the body. When an organ becomes ill or suffers from imbalance, it loses energy, and the zone where the organ is located reacts and causes the reflex point to communicate this by becoming sore. When the point is massaged, impulses are sent to the organ, which increases its energy, thus stimulating self-healing.

The concept of zone therapy is very old, although the Western therapy style dates only from the early 20th century. There is evidence that some form of zone therapy was used in China as early as 5,000 years ago, and in Egypt, depictions of reflex zones dating from around 2500 BCE have been discovered. The most prominent figure in Western reflexology was the physician William Fitzgerald, who introduced the method in the United States with his 1913 publication *Zone Therapy*. During the 1930s and 1940s, physiotherapist Eunice Ingham developed the method. She claimed that the feet were especially sensitive and that all organs could be reached via reflex points on the feet. She drew a "map" of the body on the feet and it was she who renamed the method reflexology. Modern reflexologists usually work on Ingham's theories.

Reflexology is supposed to be able to relieve a number of ailments, such as:

- Asthma, allergy, and coughing;
- Hormonal disorders;

- Skin problems and eczema;
- Headache, migraines, and other types of pain;
- Sciatica and back/neck problems;
- PMS and menopause disorders;
- Gastrointestinal disorders;
- Acute or chronic injuries;
- Sleep disorders;
- Burnout; and
- Recurring infections.

Reflexology also supposedly regulates the immune system, blood pressure, and circulation. However, reflexology has no support in evidence-based research. There are a number of studies, primarily on reflexology as a part of the treatment of MS, asthma, IBS, and cancer, but the results are contradictory. Three out of nine clinical trials showed positive effects on different ailments, but the remaining six trials did not show any positive effect at all; on the contrary, some of them showed negative effects. Two out of three trials with reflexology as treatment with the purpose of relieving pain and increasing the quality of life for palliative cancer patients only showed minor benefits, and the third trial did not show any difference at all. None of the two trials with reflexology as treatment for post-operative patients (i.e. after an operation) showed any positive effects. One article advises against reflexology treatment in connection to pregnancy, diarrhoea, vomiting, fever, inflammation in hands, feet, and ears, and inflammatory diseases, although it is unclear what the advice is based on.

To conclude, we can say that it is unclear whether reflexology is effective or not, but since some studies actually have shown negative results, it is better to try conventional massage or acupressure instead, as these treatments have documented positive effects.

Applied Kinesiology

The word kinesiology is a compound, derived from the Greek *kínesis* ("movement") and *logia* ("study"). There are two kinds of kinesiology, and they should not be confused. The first is a scientific study of human or non-human body-movement, which addresses physiological, psychological, and biomechanical movement mechanisms. It can be applied to human health, and if so, medical principles are used to analyse and improve mobility. Physiotherapists may use kinesiology for rehabilitation purposes. Scientific kinesiology is the basis for biomechanics, sports medicine, and ergonomics.

The other kind of kinesiology is the so-called applied kinesiology, which is a controversial diagnostic method. The idea behind applied kinesiology is that you can use certain muscle tests to locate imbalances, tensions, and blockages in the body's energy. By manipulating the movement apparatus (i.e. skeleton, tissue, ligaments, joints and muscles) in different ways, you can supposedly "correct" the energy system and restore balance.

In 1949, physician Robert Lovett and physiotherapists Henry and Florence Kendall presented a collection of a hundred different muscle tests. Since then, applied kinesiology has developed, especially in Europe, the United States, Canada, Australia, and New Zealand. The method was introduced in Sweden in the 1970s.

The various muscle tests used are said to be able to show deviations in different organs and in the movement apparatus, as well as malnutrition. After making the diagnosis by using the tests, the kinesiologist will recommend a treatment, which may include various massage techniques, mobilisation, stress management, relaxation techniques, nutritional therapy, or acupuncture.

There is not a lot of research on applied kinesiology. However, all available studies point in the same direction: there is no evidence that you could diagnose people through applied kinesiology, whether it concerns diseases or malnutrition. Some people claim to have been helped after being treated by a trained kinesiologist, but the research explains this with placebo. In order to get a correct diagnosis, it is important that you contact your healthcare team.

Meditation and mindfulness

Meditation has a proved positive effect on the brain. It makes us more relaxed and positive, less worried and stressed, and we also become more mindful of the present.

Positive effects from meditation have been seen in the treatment of stress, anxiety, and depression. Studies also point to a positive effect on other ailments such as obesity, high blood pressure, sleep disorders, joint pain, asthma, and eating disorders. Meditation also seems to help reduce anxiety and increase the quality of life for people with cancer and MS, and for people who have suffered a stroke.

Meditation and Mindfulness

Meditation is a way to become more mindful of the present. Some people say that it is a way for the body and soul to come into contact and find balance. Meditation is about aligning your thoughts towards a specific focal point and thus achieve personal growth, inner calm, peace of mind and a relaxed state of being. With it comes better sleep, increased knowledge of the self, reduced stress, and a strengthened immune system.

The word meditation comes from the Latin *meditare*, meaning "centring," and is actually a Western term denoting a variety of relaxation techniques. The oldest discovered descriptions of such techniques are ancient Buddhist texts written in Sanskrit, proving that meditation has been used for thousands of years. Meditation is a part of most yoga disciplines and is also intertwined with both qigong and tai chi, but you can also meditate without it being connected to any physical activity. Meditation became popular in the Western world during the 20th century. The kind of meditation known as *transcendental meditation* became very popular in the 60s when pop idols The Beatles advocated it.

There are a variety of meditation techniques, and most are based on focussing on something specific to gather your thoughts. For example, you can focus on your breathing, certain body parts, religious motifs, mantras or sounds, specific objects, or something you visualise. There is also a special chakra meditation, where you focus on one chakra at a time to balance the body's chakra energies. I will describe chakras in more detail in the next section.

Mindfulness is a relaxation technique closely related to meditation. It is about being mindful of the present and about not judging or evaluating experiences but simply observing them and letting them pass you by. In the same way, you can focus on emotions and let them pass. The idea is to train our concentration and attention, giving us a better chance to influence the one thing we *can* influence: the present. Mindfulness is supposed to help us to not dwell on the past or worry about the future. Today, mindfulness is a treatment method frequently used in Western psychotherapy.

A lot of research on meditation has been done in the West, and there is evidence of its positive effects on the brain. One interesting study was actually conducted "on commission" by the Dalai Lama, when he, in 1992, asked Western researchers to study monks while they were meditating. The study showed that meditation affects the frontal lobe of the brain in a way that makes us feel more positive and less stressed. The brain relaxes, and we may experience reduced anxiety. What happens is that the so-called neurotransmitters in the brain are affected, and there is an increase in dopamine, serotonin, and mela-tonin. To simplify, we can say that the first two substances improve our mood while melatonin causes us to relax. The amount of cortisol, which is a stress hormone, is simultaneously reduced, making us calmer. Meditation thus helps us to relax and become more positive while also being less worried and stressed, and more present in the now.

Other studies have shown that meditation has clear positive effects in the treatment of stress, anxiety, and depression. Additional studies point to positive effects on such varied ailments as obesity, high blood pressure, sleep disorders, joint pain, asthma, and eating disorders. In addition, it seems that meditation may help reduce anxiety and increase the quality of life for people with cancer and MS, as well as for people who have suffered a stroke.

One difficulty when studying the effects of meditation is that it is often intertwined with various physical therapies, such as yoga, qigong, and tai chi. That makes it difficult to determine which effects come from the medi-tation and which come from the physical activity. Perhaps the most impor-tant thing is not to determine whether it is relaxation or activity that has the largest effect (or if the effect is achieved when we find balance in our life energy), but that it is the *combination* of meditation and movement that seems so good for our health. Regardless if you believe that we humans only consist of physical building blocks or that we also have a soul or a similar body of energy, it seems good for us to strive for inner balance and harmony. It is perhaps most important for us "modern" humans, with our stress-filled lives, bad sleep, and mental disorders. That regular exercise and meditation are good for us is not really a secret; thousands of years of experience tell us that. But it is only recently that Western research and healthcare begin to tell us the same.

Chakras and Chakra Balancing

Chakras are "life wheels," or junctions in the body where alleged channels with life energy intersect. It is said that bodily functions are affected by the flow of energy through the chakras. An injury or a disease is regarded as having an effect on the energy flow. The seven major chakras are connected to various anatomical parts as well as to various emotions, and each is also associated with a certain colour.

Chakra balancing is a complementary medical treatment which is performed by a specially trained "healer" who can read the chakras of the person being treated and send in energy where it is needed to regain the balance.

There are no reliable research studies on any kind of chakra balancing as a treatment method. Whether our bodies are permeated with life energy flowing along specific channels remains unknown. But it is highly unlikely that a specially trained healer would be able to read a person's aura in order to make a medical diagnosis. To get the correct diagnosis, you should consult your healthcare team.

Chakras and Chakra Balancing

When we talk of chakras in complementary medicine, it is often the *balancing of the body's chakras* that we mean. But what are these chakras? The word is Sanskrit and means "circle" or "wheel." Hinduism and Tibetan Buddhism hold the belief that the human body contains a number of life wheels. They are not physical wheels that spin around inside us and that you could see if you looked inside, like the cogs in a robot. The life wheels instead belong to the so-called *subtle body*, which is made up of the mind, intellect and ego. The wheels are junctions where channels of life energy intersect. These channels remind us of the meridians flowing with qi energy that Taoists speak of, but in Hinduism, they are called *nadi* and the energy (as we mentioned earlier) is called *prana*. The energy primarily flows through a central channel along the spinal column, and this is where we find the seven major chakras. Each chakra governs a specific area of the body, and an injury or illness is said to affect the energy flow through the body. The body's physical and spiritual functions are also affected by the energy flow. In order to achieve bodily balance—and thereby good health—the energy must be allowed to flow freely. That is why you sometimes might need to balance your chakras.

The seven major chakras are theoretically linked to different emotions, and each is also connected to a certain colour. There is also said to be physiological connections between various anatomical parts and the locations of these chakras. Viewed from the bottom to the top, these are the seven major chakras:

- The root chakra, located at the base of the spine. It is associated with instinct, courage, safety, and security. The root chakra is said to be connected to the gonads and adrenal glands. Imbalance in this chakra manifests as problems with blood circulation, lower back pain, anger, exhaustion, or a feeling of insecurity. Colour: red.

- The sacral chakra is associated with joy of life, passion, and creativity. It is located at the root of the sexual organs, along the spine. It is said to be connected to the testicles, ovaries, and sex hormones. Imbalance in this chakra manifests as a lack of emotional control, problems in the urinary tract, sciatica, or problems in the pelvis. Colour: orange.

- The solar plexus chakra (or navel chakra) is associated with inspiration, willpower, and ambition, as well as social contact and communication. It is supposedly connected to the digestive organs. Imbalance in this chakra manifests as gastric or intestinal problems, diabetes or liver problems. Colour: yellow.

- The heart chakra is considered to be the emotional centre for the soul. It is associated with love, compassion, and harmony. It is said to be connected to the thymus, a rather small organ that is part of the immune system. The heart chakra is especially susceptible to stress, and an imbalance in it manifests as depression, problems with blood circulation, high blood pressure, heart and lung diseases, asthma, or allergy. Colour: green.

- The throat chakra is considered to be the body's centre for communication, sound, speech, and even writing. It is said to be connected to the thyroid gland, and the associated emotions include joy, trust, and forgiveness. Imbalance in this chakra manifests as stuttering or other speech problems, difficulties in expressing emotions, sore throat, goitre, cold sores, hoarseness, or neck pain. Colour: blue.

- The third-eye chakra is said to be connected to the pituitary gland, hypothalamus, and the central nervous system. It is associated with intuition, inner guidance, imagination, wisdom, and spiritual awareness. Imbalance in this chakra manifests as headache, visual impairments, ear problems, or problems with the sinuses. An imbalance here may also cause us to distrust our inner guide. Colour: indigo or deep blue.

- The crown chakra, which is located in the crown of the head, or right above it, is said to be connected to the pineal gland. This chakra is the centre for inspiration, energy, and contact with the universe. Some meditation techniques in yoga focus on the crown chakra in order to achieve a kind of meditative trance, which may be due to the connection to the pineal gland. This gland produces a hormone known as melatonin, which governs sleep, relaxation, and awakening. It is also through the crown chakra that the energy body should rise and leave the physical body when the latter dies. Imbalance in the crown chakra manifests as problems with the brain or nervous system, chronic fatigue, nervousness, or feelings of insecurity or fragmentation. Colour: white or purple.

Chakra teachings originate in Indian yogic and meditational theories, and they are very old. There is mention of chakras in 2,000-year-old Tibetan texts, but the theories have been in use for at least 4,000 years in Asia. The human body is compared to an energy receptor, and we absorb energy from every living thing around us, i.e. animals, plants and other humans, but also from the moon and the stars. There are several lesser energy centres in the body apart from the seven major chakras. Each chakra has two forces at work, one that absorbs energy and one that emits it.

So far, I have talked about the traditional theories about chakras. But there is also a more recent adaptation of the old theories, especially within the New Age movement. These newer theories claim that you can heal people by balancing their chakras in various ways, for example, by channelling the beneficial universal energy, or through vibrations, meditation, or certain crystals. It is said that each chakra is bound to different elements and special stones, as well as to certain frequencies or rhythmic vibrations. The number of spokes in the life wheels vary, and the more spokes a chakra has, the finer its frequency. Chakras are also said to be part of a so-called aura, an energy field that surrounds the body and that is visible to specially trained healers.

Chakra balancing is thus a complementary medical treatment performed by a specially trained healer who can take a reading of a person's chakras and then deliver the appropriate amount of energy needed to balance the chakras. After the treatment, it is recommended that you take some time to relax and talk through and process the impressions.

Another form of chakra balancing is connected with yoga, respiratory training, and sound therapy (we take a closer look at sound therapy in Chapter 6). In this treatment, you use different sounds, such as mantras and vocal toning, to balance the body's chakras. The vibrations of the sounds are said to be the balancing factor. Sometimes, sighs and yawns are also used as these are said to be a natural way for the body to release tension. The sounds are often combined with simpler yoga exercises and deep breathing.

There are no reliable scientific studies on any kind of chakra balancing as a treatment method. Whether our bodies are perfused with life energy through meridians, nadi, some other means, or not at all is yet to be discovered. But I find it highly unlikely that a specially trained healer could read a person's aura to diagnose diseases. Meditation, yoga, and qigong have been proven effective as treatments for certain ailments, whether you believe in chakras or not, but in order to receive the correct diagnosis you should always consult your health-care team.

Crystal Therapy

Crystal healing, crystal therapy, or gem therapy is a form of treatment where the aim is to balance the body's energy by placing or fastening different crystals on the skin. The idea behind this is that different rocks and gemstones emit different frequencies or vibrations depending on their colour, and that these frequencies can harmonise the body's energy. The crystals are said to absorb light and then project it into our bodies, where it affects our energy aura in various ways. Crystals may also be used to balance the body's chakras. They are then placed on those parts of the body where the chakras are projected. The Swedish trade union KAM (the Committee for Alternative Medicine) has presented a chart displaying which body part is harmonised by which crystal colour:

Energy	Colour of crystal	Body part that is harmonised
Wind	Green	Liver, gallbladder, muscles, tendons, joints
Warmth	Red	Heart, small intestine, arteries, veins
Heat	Orange	Brain, spinal cord, nerves, endocrine glands
Moisture	Yellow	Stomach, spleen, pancreas, fatty tissue, lymph
Aridity	White, brown	Lungs, colon, mucous membranes, skin, immune system
Cold	Blue, black	Urinary bladder, kidneys, urinary tract, skeleton, genitals

Almost all cultures around the world hold some beliefs that crystals and rocks possess special powers. Quartz in its various forms (onyx, citrine, and amethyst are all varieties of quartz) is regarded in crystal therapy as especially potent in its ability to enhance the rhythmic vibrations in the life energy, counteract stress and strengthen the resistance towards diseases. It is true that quartz has the ability to vibrate on a certain frequency, which makes it useful in radio equipment and clockwork. However, there is no scientific evidence of quartz or any other crystal or rock having therapeutic properties. On the contrary, geologists claim that rocks lack such properties. In fact, there is nothing special about quartz, which is the second most common mineral in the Earth's crust. It exists everywhere around us in various forms: as minute grains in sand and rock; in gravel and concrete; or as "gemstones," like amethysts, tiger's eyes, or agates. There is no significant difference in chemical composition between, for example, a white quartz and a black smoky quartz. The difference in colour comes from minor differences in the pressure and heat when the rock was formed, and from various impurities or traces of metal present in the rock. Thus, we are not talking about different gemstones with different properties, as you may sometimes hear the vendors claim when they sell the stones at high prices.

From a modern scientific and medical point of view, it is highly unlikely that you could cure diseases by having stones placed on your body. But since a placebo sometimes can have as much an effect as any other treatment method, it is not impossible that crystal therapy can benefit you, as long as you believe in the treatment and your condition does not need a better evidence-based treatment or immediate medical attention.

Various Forms of Healing

The idea behind healing is that people can promote good health, cure diseases, and improve personal growth through certain thought patterns and rituals. This form of belief has existed for as long as humans have, regardless of geographical origin, religion, or culture.

There is no reliable research supporting the claims about healing. There are, however, studies indicating that spirituality in the form of prayer, pilgrimages, spiritual healing, and the like can have an effect on certain ailments. The researchers claim that this is due to the placebo effect. There are also studies indicating that religious psychotherapy can have positive effects on anxiety and depression.

4 Various Forms of Healing

As we have now touched on healing, it is time to move on and describe in more detail a couple of different forms of healing treatments. The term *healing* can be confusing since it can mean all forms of curing or medical progression, for example, when you say that your broken leg is healing. But in complementary medicine, the word is a collective term denoting various treatment methods based on strengthening a person's spirituality and spiritual health. The idea behind healing is that people can promote health, cure illnesses, and favour personal growth through certain thought patterns and rituals. This form of belief has existed for as long as humans have, regardless of geographical origin, religion or culture. There are many different forms of healing, such as spiritual healing, reconnecting, Reiki, shamanistic healing, trance, crystal, angel, and animal healing. In a moment, we will take a closer look at two of these, reiki and shamanism, but first, I would like to briefly describe the theory upon which many of the modern healing methods are based.

In the beginning of the 20th century, American mystic Edgar Cayce (1877-1945) claimed that each individual emits a certain vibration as a result of the condition of that individual's body, mind, and soul. Emotional disorders as well as pathogenic factors create vibrations that differ from the individual's fundamental vibration. This causes disturbances in the nervous system. Many forms of healing are based on the belief that all matter consists of vibrating atoms, and that the human body emits a certain vibration that begins in each cell and organ. The interplay between atoms, the human body, and the surroundings cause a certain tension, which in turn creates a certain mental mood. The interplay between the body's organs, the mind's thoughts, and the mental mood in turn create what is called *energy*. Healers claim that this energy flows through the body along certain paths (some equate these paths to *nadi* and claim that the energy is gathered in chakras). Through rituals and special methods to align the thoughts, the healer tries to bring about a change in the vibrations in the person receiving treatment. The healer also often tries to harmonise the body's living tissue with the creative energy and increase blood flow in epidermis and hypodermis. This supposedly resolves energy blockages, restores a healthy energy flow, creates a sense of wellbeing, and restores the balance between body, mind, and soul. The result of this is that the body's own ability to self-heal increases. Although these vibrations were not described by Cayce until the 20th century, many ancient forms of healing have a similar basic belief in people's inherent energy and its interplay with the surroundings. As we have seen, this idea is also fundamental in more physically oriented treatment methods like yoga, qigong, and acupuncture.

There is no good quality research that supports the claims behind the art of healing, neither regarding the beneficial effects nor the underlying theories about the body's vibrations. However, there are studies suggesting that spirituality in the form of prayer, pilgrimages, spiritual healing, and similar religious methods (regardless of religion) may be effective against certain ailments, although researchers say that this is due to the placebo effect, as we mentioned in Chapter 2. There are also studies suggesting that religious psychotherapy may have positive effects on anxiety and depression.

Reiki

Reiki is a Japanese form of healing. The word means something like "universal life energy." The method contains various rituals and symbols. Researchers have not been able to prove the alleged effects of these rituals and symbols, but as with other forms of healing, the placebo effect should not be overlooked. However, if you need to be diagnosed or if you suffer from a serious disease, it is important that you contact your healthcare team.

Reiki

I will let the Japanese form of healing known as Reiki be an example of what a more ritualistic healing method may look like. Reiki can be viewed as a form of *laying on of hands*, that is, when a therapist puts his/her hands on the person receiving treatment for the purpose of transferring spiritual or healing energy. However, Reiki can also be given as distance treatment.

The word *reiki* consists of two Japanese words: *rei* (the meaning of which is difficult to translate, but can be described as a "higher intelligence," "universal spirit," or "divine awareness"), and *ki* (which is the Japanese word for the life energy qi). Put together, the term *reiki* means something like "divine energy," although that does not quite capture all it encompasses. In 1922, Usui Mikao founded the first Reiki association and opened a clinic in Tokyo. According to the Swedish Reiki Association, the method "came to" Usui Mikao when he suffered a crisis in life. During a course of treatment at the Buddhist temple on Mount Kurama, Reiki supposedly "came to him," and he received incredible healing powers. However, he might also have developed the method from his own experiences of Buddhism and *kiko* (the Japanese version of qigong). Regardless of how it was developed, he gave Reiki healing to a large number of people after the great earthquake that devastated Tokyo in 1923. The demand was so great that he opened a larger clinic. He eventually became famous all over Japan as a great healer. A number of followers with similar stories of life crises, sickness, and healing broke away from the basic teachings and created methods of their own. With time, these methods have been adapted to Western culture and spread to Europe and the United States. The International Center for Reiki Training (ICRT) was founded by the American William Lee Rand, and he is credited with making Reiki available to the public in the West.

Reiki is a philosophy and a method that is divided into different levels that you achieve one after the other, similar to martial arts, where you win belts of different colours according to the rank you achieve as you learn more advanced techniques. The first level in Reiki is called *Shoden* or simply

Reiki I. The focus here is to use a certain number of hand positions to primarily heal yourself, but also others. You also want to deepen your contact with the Reiki energy through special meditation techniques. This level of Reiki healing cannot be given as distance therapy, and you do not use any of the special symbols used in higher levels. The second level is called *Okuden* or *Reiki II.* This level also includes hand positions, but the focus is now on different kinds of distance treatments. Special symbols are used for this purpose (see below). People who have mastered Reiki II can provide healing on the physical, emotional, and mental levels, both through laying on of hands and distance therapy. The third and highest level is called *Shinpiden, Reiki III,* or the *Master Level.* Here, the practitioner's skills are further honed through "initiation" from a Master who draws secret and holy Reiki symbols, helping the practitioner open up to the Reiki energy so that he/she can use it in new ways.

Different kinds of healing have different kinds of rituals and symbols. Here, I let Reiki exemplify what it may look like. In Reiki, practitioners primarily use the following five symbols:

Choku Rei – This is a symbol for power and by drawing it and speaking its name three times out loud or in your mind, you increase the Reiki effect (which is about projecting the surrounding energy to wherever you want). This symbol is used at the beginning and end of a treatment, but it is also used during sessions to reinforce other symbols, for protection or to cleanse the area of negative energies. It can also be used to make a wish come true.

Sei Hei Ki – This is a mental and emotional symbol said to assist in clearing away negative thoughts and emotional blockages, achieving inner peace and harmony, and balancing the right and left hemispheres of the brain. This symbol is especially useful against various forms of addiction.

Hon Sha Ze Sho Nen – This is a symbol for distance that is used in distance healing but also when looking back into the past or forward into the future. It is also used when initiating others into Reiki from a distance.

Tamarasha – This is a symbol for balance used when balancing the body's energy and, in certain forms of Reiki, the body's chakras. You begin by balancing the root chakra, since balanced energy will then flow upwards to the next chakra, and so on. A chakra thus receives energy from the one closest below it. The crown chakra, at the top, is regarded as being in direct contact with the universe and the universal energy. This balancing symbol is also used for relieving pain and to initiate a practitioner in more advanced levels.

Dai Ko Mio – This is the most powerful symbol in the original Reiki method, and it is called the Master symbol. It is only used by those initiated into the Master level. The symbol is said to be able to heal the soul and cure illnesses. It can also provide inner peace, personal growth, and be a guide on the way to enlightenment.

Only a handful of studies exploring the effects of Reiki healing have been published. A systematic review from 2008 drew the conclusion that the value of Reiki cannot be proved. The same goes for most other similar methods of healing, but as I stated earlier, the placebo effect should not be overlooked. However, if you need to be diagnosed, or you suffer from a serious disease, it is very important that you contact your healthcare team.

Shamanism

Shamanism exists all over the world and probably originates from the time when humans were hunters and gatherers and when nature played a more immediate role for us than it does in our modern society. Today, shamanism is more prevalent among aboriginal peoples than among urban populations. The basic concept of all shamanism is that nature is animate, that it has a soul or is made up of gods and spirits living in plants, rocks, and watercourses. All parts of the universe are regarded as connected to each other through energies and vibrations. There are also different planes of existence that are connected to each other; for example, the dream plane and the "ordinary" plane. Our "ordinary" world is often viewed as an illusion while the spirit world is the place from where everything is being controlled. You might think of it as a puppet show where the puppets (we humans and all other creatures in the "ordinary" world) are being controlled by forces (spirits) in the spirit world.

A shaman, witch doctor, druid, or medicine man, is a person who, by entering a trance, can travel between the different planes of existence or communicate with the spirits to achieve knowledge, for example, in order to cure illnesses. The word shaman originally comes from the Siberian language Evenki and means "one who knows." It signifies a person who comprehends the mysteries of life and death. Shamans in different cultures have different names and their own special rituals, but the basic idea described above is a common denominator for most of them. These are a few of the different types of shamans around the world:

- Native American medicine men;
- Sami noaidi;
- African medicine men;
- Hawaiian kahunas;
- Celtic druids and priestesses;
- Caribbean witch doctors;
- Siberian shamans;
- Indigenous South American shamans;
- Ancient Turkish/Hungarian/Mongolian Tengrian shamans; and
- Old Norse practitioners of *seiðr* (a type of sorcery).

Shamans hold a high position in society, as our European priests used to do (and still do in some countries). It is the task of the shaman to guide the tribe and, primarily, to act as healer. A shaman can also be responsible for guiding the spirits of the dead to the land of the dead. If these spirits do not arrive there, they will remain in this world as ghosts.

Symbols are very important in shamanism. Native American totems come to mind, perhaps. Animal totems are important symbols used by many indigenous peoples. Another recurring symbol is the Tree of Life, a tree that links all the worlds or planes of existence and that encloses the universe. Two examples of such trees are Yggdrasil of the Old Norse religion and Wacah Chan of the ancient Mayan culture. The Tree of Life is a representation of what is usually called the *axis mundi*, the world axis, which is an axis that penetrates creation and connects the Earth, the underworld, and the heavens. In many cultures, this axis is represented by a tree, but in other cultures, it can be a mountain, a pillar, a pyramid, or something else. A third important symbol in many shamanistic rituals is the drum. The drum helps the shaman enter a trance, and it can also have special symbols painted or carved on it, like on the Sami noaidic drums.

When the shaman has entered a trance, he or she can embark on a "journey" through the different planes of existence. The journey is always undertaken for a specific purpose, usually to perform a certain task such as counteract a disease, understand the nature of broken taboos, find a lost or tormented soul, help restore the balance between different levels of the cosmos, or reduce the gap between the spirit world and the tribe. Shamanism is different from spiritism in that the journey to the spirit world is an active one, while spiritism involves conjuring spirits to our world. In spiritistic experiences in Haitian voodoo or ecstatic dancing, the medium does not recall his or her visionary experiences. Shamans, on the other hand, are fully aware of the ecstasy and take full responsibility for what happens during the vision quest. Shamans use a number of means to help them in their work:

> **A supernatural force or spirit who helps the shaman** – A spirit of a person or an animal can be summoned to guide the shaman in his/her task or act as guardian or helper.

> **Ceremonies and rituals** – Various ceremonies and rituals are used by shamans of different cultures to make contact with an inner reality or to penetrate the different cosmic dimensions.

> **The drum** – Drumming is a means of focussing the shaman's awareness. The even, monotonous rhythm evokes brainwaves within the theta frequency, 4-7 hertz. These brainwaves are associated with deep meditation and sleep. Shamans describe their trance experiences as a waking dream, real experiences in the dimension where they take place, and not as hallucinations or fantasies.

Singing and dancing – Enhances mental focus through controlled breathing and monotonous movements. Among the medicine men of Cuba, dancing is regarded as the most important method for getting in touch with primal instincts and make them visible. The ritual known as *toque de santo* or the "feast of the gods" contains ancient songs of African origin accompanied by a rhythmic pattern of drumming. The participants dance freely, and eventually, in an unplanned way, they make room for the person who has been "chosen by the gods" to be the centre of the ritual at that time. The entire affair can be perceived as an out-of-body experience. Dancing is an important element of the mystic experiences in Sufism as well. Perhaps you have seen the characteristically spinning Dervish dancers in their long white garments.

Scent and taste – The scents created by boiling herbal mixtures with essential oils are used in many spiritualistic healing traditions. Perfume, tobacco, and other things are also common. Stimulating the senses in this way seems to enhance the biochemical parts of the process of entering an altered state of consciousness. However, it is not only in shamanistic rituals that scent and taste are used to stimulate the spirit. Consider, for example, Catholic ceremonies where incense is often used, and at Communion, everybody tastes wafers and wine—symbols of the body and blood of Christ.

Psychotropic substances – By using certain hallucinogenic substances that affect the central nervous system, shamans can alter their state of consciousness and thereby enter a trance. However, rhythmic music alone usually suffices.

To the shaman, there is no difference between what others perceive as "real" and "unreal" worlds. Some psychologists have described the phenomenon as similar to near-death experiences or out-of-body experiences. This suggests that our consciousness could be an expression of a function that is not necessarily connected to the physical reality. There is a lot of research being conducted on the shamanistic state of trance, and it will be interesting to see the results.

Most shamans and medicine men have great knowledge of medicinal plants, and we know that these can be effective in certain contexts. Many of the active substances in our modern pharmaceuticals come from plants, and the Amazon rainforest is a veritable treasure chest. This takes us to the next chapter, which deals with herbal medicine.

Natural Remedies and Health Food

Originally, all medicine was based on natural substances, mainly medicinal plants. Around 1920, a systematisation was initiated, and standardised pharmaceuticals quickly replaced the old natural remedies. Many common drugs, such as aspirin and morphine, can trace their origins to various plants.

Many people have a basic belief that whatever is natural is good and that diseases can be prevented by using natural products. In one study from 2012, it was shown that 52 percent of Americans (approximately 150 million people) spent 5.5 billion dollars on various health products. In Europe, sales had already reached that level by 2003. In Germany, many such products are completely or partially included in the pharmaceutical benefits scheme.

The information available about the products and their potential side effects is often insufficient. In one report from the United States, it was shown that 32 percent of plant-based products were made from plant parts that did not even contain the substances that were supposed to be the active substances.

Several natural food supplements have been shown to contain harmful substances. Despite this, they are still on the market. One example is zeolite-based preparations that are marketed as detox products.

5 Natural Remedies and Health Foods

We have now come to another area in complementary medicine: natural remedies. Originally, all medicines were based on natural products, especially medicinal plants, but nowadays many pharmaceuticals are produced synthetically. There are also semi-synthetic pharmaceuticals, which means that the basis is natural substances which are then somewhat modified. Around 1920, a systematisation of plant-based medicines was initiated, and standardised pharmaceuticals quickly replaced the old natural remedies. Many common drugs, such as aspirin, morphine, and prednisolone can trace their origins to various plants. But it is not these standardised and originally plant-based pharmaceuticals that we mean when we talk about natural remedies in complementary medicine. Rather, it is herbal medicines and health foods that are being marketed as health-promoting or curatives without having been through the rigorous research and testing that is a requirement for standardised pharmaceuticals. In this chapter, I want to highlight the side effects that these natural remedies can have and also mention a few of the most common remedies that are marketed as proven effective. We will also take a closer look at three specific areas within the world of natural remedies: Bach flower remedies, homeopathy, and anthroposophic medicine.

Many people still have a basic belief that whatever is natural is good, and that diseases can be prevented by using natural products. In some cases, this is true, in some cases not. However, this basic belief has created a huge market for health products, and in many countries, voids in government legislation are used by companies to sell products that have not been sufficiently tested and sometimes are harmful instead of healthy. Since the food industry has significantly lower control requirements than the pharmaceutical industry, many of the products can be sold in grocery stores or together with beauty care products. In the United States, *cosmeceuticals* (*cosmetics* + *pharmaceuticals*) have become a huge industry where consumers are led to believe that certain bioactive elements in the products will have a number of different effects that promote both good health and beauty. In many cases, there are not enough studies to prove any such effects.

The market for health foods and natural remedies is enormous. In a survey from 2012, conducted by the National Health and Nutrition Examination Survey, 52 percent of Americans used some form of health product (vitamins, minerals or plant-based). This means approximately 150 million people in the United States alone. Health products sales reached 5.5 billion dollars. In Europe, sales had already reached that level by 2003 and have only increased since then. The most common health products include fish oil, probiotics and prebiotics, glucosamine, echinacea (coneflower), Arctic root, St John's wort, cranberries, garlic, ginseng, and gingko biloba. In Sweden, some of the most common products supposedly strengthen the immune system or have a stimulating effect, but the best-sellers are food supplements and vitamins. Other commonly sold products aim at general health, weight loss, joint pain and eye health. In Germany, to give another example, a large proportion of the population uses natural remedies (60 percent according to one report), and many such products are completely or partially included in the pharmaceutical benefits scheme.

So, huge quantities of health products and natural remedies are available— but do they work? It is difficult to say, and it can differ a great deal between different products. Most studies are of poor quality, and in addition, there are often no follow-up studies that examine how the products correspond to consumer expectations. There are no official requirements or demands from the authorities for such studies to be made. There is no five-year report like there is for pharmaceuticals, and no such report is necessary for companies to get permission to market products. Nor is it necessary to present information about the pharmacodynamic properties of the products, that is, how they break down in the human body and how they interact with other health products, foods, or pharmaceuticals. Systematic reports about suspected or confirmed side effects are usually not published. All this means that you, as a consumer, are often not given enough information about the products or their potential side effects. I am not saying that the production and marketing of natural remedies and health foods are completely without regulations. In Europe, a 2004 directive from the European Union governs the registration of health foods that contain plant extracts. This directive states that any company that wishes to register a product must be able to prove that whatever is said in the marketing of that product regarding its safety and effectiveness is true. The company that registers the product must also do a follow-up of the marketing campaign as well as report any serious side effects. Despite these requirements, it is still a partially unregulated market that we consumers enter.

There are several factors that affect both the side effects and the desired effects in a remedy: the raw materials and parts of the plants used, how the raw materials are stored, and how the remedies are produced. One report from the United States showed that 32 percent of plant-based products were made of plant parts that did not contain any of the substances that were supposed to be the active substances. Other reports have showed that products marketed as "natural" actually contained conventional drugs. Not only is this false marketing, it is also potentially very dangerous if these products are combined with other pharmaceuticals. Products with unacceptable levels of lead, mercury, or arsenic have also been marketed. It is thus extremely important that you do your research before you "botanize" among the natural remedies.

Some of the active substances in natural remedies and health food products may affect hormone metabolism, blood pressure, and brain activity. UpToDate is a database that collects evidence-based facts about various pharmaceuticals, natural remedies, and diagnoses as well as treatment principles for various diseases and ailments. Here, you can find certain facts about how conventional drugs interact with natural remedies. One example is that garlic may react with antidiabetics, and it is therefore important for diabetics to know this. Other examples include liquorice root, which affects blood pressure, and gingko biloba that may react with blood thinners. If you have a diagnosis, suffer from any ailment or are already using pharmaceuticals, it is very important that you consult your healthcare team before you try different natural remedies.

Now that we have talked so much about side effects and insufficient regulations, it might sound as if there is nothing good in natural remedies. That, however, is not the case. As I mentioned earlier in this chapter, many of our standardised pharmaceuticals are based on natural substances, and herbal medicines have always been a part of man kind's fight against diseases. In fact, close to 80 percent of the world's population uses treatments that do not belong to evidence-based medicine. Many of these treatments are based on various herbal remedies. There are studies suggesting that some natural remedies have positive effects. Below, I briefly list some of the more common.

- Fish oil (omega-3) – Fatty acids from fat fish (such as salmon, herring, and mackerel) counteract blood clots and make the blood vessels smooth. Fish oil has been approved as a medicine in Norway. Studies indicate that fish oil may also have positive effects in children with ADHD. It should not be used if you already use blood thinners.
- Probiotics – "Good" bacteria that balance the intestinal flora. It may prevent traveller's diarrhoea, i.e. when the intestinal flora is not used to the bacterial flora present in a new location. Also available as food supplement.
- Garlic – In folk medicine, garlic is a classic remedy against colds, and it has also traditionally been used against atherosclerosis and to lower cholesterol levels. If you are using blood thinners, you should be careful with garlic. The same goes if you are a diabetic.
- Echinacea (coneflower) – Marketed as a remedy for relieving cold symptoms, but it is important to take it at the right time—when the cold is about to break out. It then supposedly relieves the symptoms and shortens the time that the cold lasts. Coneflower belongs to the daisy family of flowers, and if you are allergic to those plants, you should not use echinacea.
- St John's wort – Studies have shown some effect against depression and anxiety. Although some studies have compared the effects of St John's wort with conventional antidepressants, there is no basis for general recommendations. Due to the fact that St John's wort tends to interact with other pharmaceuticals, it should not be combined with these. St John's wort may also block the effect of birth control pills and heart medications.

- Cranberries – May protect the mucous membranes in the urinary tract against bacteria. Some consumers believe that cranberries relieve and help prevent urinary tract infections if you eat the berries raw or drink cranberry juice. However, clinical studies which may form a basis for general recommendations are lacking.
- Ginseng – A so called "adaptogen" that is said to enhance performance and increase the cells' oxygen consumption. Adaptogens are biological substances that are said to affect us (e.g. by direct cell stimulation) in ways that enable us to better handle negative factors in our surroundings, such as stress. There is not enough clinical research to warrant an approval of adaptogens by the evidence-based healthcare system. Ginseng is also used against fatigue and for strengthening the immune system. It should be avoided by patients using blood thinners.
- Ginkgo biloba – Some studies show that the leaves of this tree may increase blood circulation and be effective in the treatment of memory disorders, concentration problems, fatigue, and dizziness in the elderly – but UpToDate advises against these uses. In particular, gingko biloba should be avoided by anyone using blood thinners.
- Zinc – Available as lozenges against bad breath since zinc binds the sulphurous substances that sometimes cause the bad breath.
- Folic acid – Available as a food supplement and is recommended to pregnant women since it reduces the risk of spina bifida in the foetus. Folic acid is a vitamin B that is necessary for the body's ability to produce blood. It exists naturally in yeast, raw vegetables, meat, and liver.
- Calcium – Calcium exists naturally in dairy products and is also available as food supplement. It prevents osteoporosis.

I would also like to highlight one "warning example," that is, a natural supplement that has been proven to contain harmful substances but is still being sold – zeolite-based detox. Zeolites are minerals that mainly contain silicon dioxide (also known as silica) and aluminium oxide. There are many forms of zeolites, some natural and some synthetic. They form naturally when volcanic minerals and ash react with alkaline groundwater. Because of this, zeolite-based food supplements are sometimes marketed as volcanic sand or volcanic ash. Zeolites are also found in beauty care products. The chemical properties and structure of zeolites enable them to trade their ions for those of other substances, thus binding heavy metals and other substances. This makes them valuable in the chemical industry, for example, as purification filters and water softeners.

But why are zeolites marketed as food supplements? Well, the idea is the same as in the chemical industry: that the zeolites will cleanse the body by binding harmful substances. Zeolite-based products are sold as colon cleansers or detox. The recommendation might say that you should mix 20 grams of zeolites with 10 grams of gastrointestinal stimulants in water and consume it two to three times a day for a period of two to three days. This is said to clear out any harmful substances, but the risk is that the opposite occurs. Some zeolite-based products contain hazardous levels of lead, arsenic, and dioxins. This came to the attention of the Swedish Food Administration as early as 2002. Lead can cause damage to the nervous system. Foetuses and small children are particularly sensitive, so children and pregnant women are especially sensitive to high levels of lead. (That is why pregnant women should not eat fish from lakes, which often contain elevated levels of heavy metals.) Arsenic and dioxins are both considered carcinogenic (cancer-causing), and dioxins impair the immune system. The reported side effects connected with zeolite-based products include abdominal pain, nausea, vomiting, coughing, memory disorders, and cancer spread. Abnormal blood values have also been reported, for example, elevated levels of heavy metals in the blood and low levels of potassium ions. There are reports showing positive effects from zeolite-based products as colon cleansers. However, these reports have been published by companies that market the products, and therefore cannot be trusted. The reports also lack scientific evidence.

While working on this book, I have also worked on a compilation reviewing the most common risks and benefits of the best-selling health food products. The compilation is currently under publication.

Bach Flower Remedies, Homeopathy, and Anthroposophic Medicine

While modern science aims to examine the active substances in various plants, there are a number of specific traditions within herbal medicine that explain the remedies' effects rather differently. These traditions have other theories as to why the natural remedies are effective and how they work. I will now present three of these traditions.

Bach Flower Remedies

In the 1930s, British physician Edward Bach (pronounced "batch") developed a treatment method designed to heal people by using essences from various flowers to treat their emotional condition. Bach worked at the London Homeopathic Hospital and was thus influenced by the homeopathic healing tradition (I will describe homeopathy in more detail below). The new flower remedies did not contain any plant parts, only what Bach referred to as the flowers' "energy," dissolved in water and alcohol. Systematic and clinical studies have not been able to prove any effect beyond placebo for these flower remedies.

The basic idea behind the remedies was that the human body reflects mental imbalances through physical and functional problems. Once you realise what the fundamental disharmony is and what the cause is, you can be healed. The flower remedies are said to affect emotions and moods in order to restore mental balance and promote healing. The idea was not entirely new; in the 16th century, Swiss alchemist and physician Paracelsus worked with dew drops from plants on a similar basis. Bach's method is also closely related to aroma therapy, which has been used in various forms for millennia (I will describe aroma therapy in the next chapter).

Bach flower remedies (or BFRs) are still on the market today. They are sold all over the world but are most common in Europe and the United States. All production is still taking place at a specific centre outside Oxford in England. There are 38 flower remedies in Bach's original set. They are listed below with their proposed properties and English and Latin names:

Agrimony (*Agrimonia eupatoria*): For restless people who often escape problems and conflicts—and perhaps deaden them with alcohol or drugs. Supposedly increases independency and the ability to show emotions and view problems objectively. Also, it supposedly reduces the inclination to escape problems through substance abuse.

Aspen (*Populus tremula*): For people who feel vague fear without a clear cause, perhaps in combination with nightmares. This essence supposedly gives a person the courage to face that fear and also brings more joy in life.

Beech (*Fagus sylvatica*): For intolerant and critical people who lack humility and find it difficult to accept shortcomings in other people. The essence supposedly helps develop a tolerance for other people and increases respect for the opinions of others.

Centaury *(Centaurium erthraea)*: For shy people and people who have difficulties setting boundaries or saying no. The essence supposedly increases the ability to set boundaries and boosts a sense of self.

Cerato *(Ceratostigma willmottiana)*: For people who tend to imitate others and excessively ask for advice, and for people who go against their own convictions in order to heed the advice of others. This essence supposedly increases your intuitive ability, making you trust your own inner voice more often.

Cherry plum *(Prunus cerasifera)*: For those who feel desperation and fear of losing control, becoming violent, or worst of all, committing suicide. The energy from the cherry blossoms supposedly creates an inner force, courage, sanity, and strength so that you may regain control.

Chestnut bud *(Aesculus hippocastanum)*: For inattentive people who repeat the same mistakes and accidents. These drops are supposed to provide mental flexibility and improved learning capacity, as well as increased ability for self-reflection.

Chicory *(Cichorium intybus)*: For selfish people and people who display a dominating kind of love. It is also supposed to help children who constantly crave attention. Supposedly, chicory provides the ability to feel unconditional love and express care without being demanding.

Clematis *(Clematis vitalba)*: For daydreamers who escape to their own world when faced with problems. Also for people with memory problems and people who are often sleepy or tired. This essence supposedly gives an increased interest in life and one's surroundings. It's also said to enhance concentration, presence of mind, and memory.

Crab apple *(Malus pumila)*: For people who feel a sense of self-loathing, have negative thoughts about themselves, or feel impure. This can manifest itself in excessive cleanliness, fear of bacteria, and cleaning mania. This essence is said to help you put things into perspective and accept yourself, which lets you get rid of the obsessive cleanliness behaviour and affirm yourself.

Elm *(Ulmus procera)*: Should be used when you suddenly become overwhelmed with duties that you do not feel capable of performing, or for temporary feelings of inadequacy. The essence supposedly helps you overcome these feelings and regain confidence.

Gentian *(Gentiana amarella)*: For sceptical, doubting, and pessimistic people who easily lose heart. The essence is supposed to help you see the positive in every situation, be less influenced by setbacks, and feel confident in the face of adversity.

Gorse *(Ulex europaeus)*: For people who feel depressed or have given up hope. Supposedly, gorse gives new hope and the realisation that you have the ability to make your situation better.

Heather *(Calluna vulgaris)*: For self-absorbed people who are poor listeners and instead talk about their own problems all the time. Heather is said to reduce the egotism, increase the ability to listen to others, and help develop empathy for other people's problems.

Holly *(Ilex aquifolium)*: Said to help against all forms of hatred, jealousy, envy, and suspiciousness. This essence supposedly increases the ability to feel joy for other people's success and feel unconditional love.

Honeysuckle *(Lonicera caprifolium)*: Helps reduce nostalgia and homesickness; also for people who are over-attached to the past and cannot leave it. This essence is supposed to help you live in the present and move on in life.

Hornbeam *(Carpinus betulus)*: For people who feel that they do not have sufficient strength to cope with everyday life, postpone things or feel fatigue and loss of energy. These drops are said to make you more alert, as well as provide will-power and the ability to take initiative.

Impatiens *(Impatiens glandulifera)*: For impatient people who do everything quickly and cannot tolerate the slowness of other people, impatiens supposedly gives increased patience and calm.

Larch *(Larix decidua)*: For people with a lack of confidence or who often feel inferior to others. This essence is supposed to make you more determined and give increased confidence.

Mimulus *(Mimulus guttatus)*: For people with various phobias of known things, such as darkness, flying, and diseases; also for shy people. These drops are said to reduce hypersensitivity and give courage, trust, and a larger appetite for life.

Mustard *(Sinapis arvensis)*: Used to treat melancholia and depression that has no obvious cause. Mustard is said to provide inner stability, faith in the future, and increased happiness.

Oak *(Quercus robur)*: For people who work too much and are unable to stop. These drops are said to increase the ability to delegate tasks, lower the demands for your own performance, and help you listen to your body's signals so that you quit in time.

Olive *(Olea europaea)*: For those who feel completely exhausted and cannot find any joy in things that previously brought satisfaction, or for those who do not have time for pleasures and relaxation. Olive is said to restore strength, vitality, and inner peace, and increase stamina.

Pine *(Pinus sylvestris)*: For people who feel unworthy and guilty. The pine essence is said to provide the ability to affirm oneself and thereby embrace life.

Red chestnut *(Aesculus carnea)*: For people who are overly concerned with the wellbeing of others and who always assume the worst. Red chestnut supposedly strengthens the ability to keep calm under pressure and express positive thoughts to those who need them.

Rock rose *(Rosa canina)*: Used against apathy, chronic fatigue, and feelings of emptiness. This essence is supposed to provide energy and enthusiasm for life as well as increase motivation and vitality.

Rock water *("Aqua petra")*: This is not a plant essence, but simply water from a rocky stream. People who live very strictly and dismissively are supposedly helped by this essence to relax and become more open and generous towards themselves and others.

Scleranthus *(Scleranthus annuus)*: For indecisive people and people whose mood swings often between extremes. This essence is said to increase concentration and determination.

Star of Bethlehem *(Ornithogalum umbellatum)*: Used with accidents of different kinds, as well as against shock and trauma. Star of Bethlehem is said to neutralise shock and restore harmony to body and soul by resolving blockages in the energy flow caused by the shock.

Sweet chestnut *(Castanea sativa)*: Used against extreme anxiety and despair; also for those who have no hope for the future. Sweet chestnut supposedly provides inner calm and spiritual harmony.

Vervain *(Verbena officinalis)*: For high-strung people and those who suffer from insomnia. Vervain is said to make you more alert to the body's signals telling you it needs rest. It is also supposed to reduce mental and physical strains and provide better sleep.

Vine *(Vitis vinifera)*: For dominant and power-hungry people who may lack compassion. This essence is said to develop humility and empathy so that you better understand other people and may use your authority in a beneficial way.

Walnut *(Juglans regia)*: Supposedly useful when you face major changes in life, such as career changes, divorce, relocation, etc., as well as physical changes such as puberty, menopause, pregnancy, etc. This essence is supposed to help you break old patterns and better adapt to new situations.

Water violet *(Hottonia palustris)*: For reserved people who prefer to draw back and dislike the involvement of other people. Water violet is said to help you act humbly and humanely, as well as better enjoy the company of others.

White chestnut *(Aesculus hippocastanum)*: For people who cannot shut out certain thoughts and who have trouble sleeping because of their thoughts. This essence is supposed to provide inner calm and make you aware of your ability to control your thoughts.

Wild oat *(Bromus ramosus)*: For people who cannot decide what they want in life or have trouble finding their mission. This essence supposedly provides clarity regarding ambitions, talents, and possibilities so that you may find your place in life.

Wild rose *(Helianthemum nummularium)*: This essence is said to help against dread, panic attacks, nightmares, and muscle tension caused by fear or anxiety, by increasing your courage and resolving extreme states of tension.

Willow *(Salix vitellina)*: For people who feel bitterness and self-pity; also for pessimists and people incapable of feeling gratitude. This essence is said to give the ability to see yourself and your role in a larger context. It supposedly also makes it easier to forgive others and feel joy for their success.

There is also a so-called *Rescue Remedy*, which is a mix of Star of Bethlehem, rock rose, impatiens, cherry plum, and clematis. It is supposed to be used in a crisis and against severe stress, or when you feel strong fear or panic. Studies have examined this mixture, but the results indicate no effect at all. Bach flower remedies are considered free of side effects, but it is unclear what the effects might be if they are combined with conventional pharmaceuticals, so it is always wise to consult your healthcare team prior to testing them.

Homeopathy

Homeopathy is a controversial and debated complementary medical method. The method is difficult to assess systematically and objectively since homeopathy is based on each patient being treated in an individual manner. Homeopathy rests on the principle that like cures like, i.e. that the same substance that causes disease symptoms in a healthy individual will cure the disease in one who is ill.

Despite massive criticism from researchers and medical staff, homeopathy continues to be popular, especially in Europe but also in North America and Asia.

There are a few reports showing negative effects, especially for homeopathic preparations in detox and weight loss. Given the current lack of research and many health authorities' negative attitude towards homeopathy, patients should not use homeopathic preparations for any medical condition for which there is a better evidence-based alternative.

Homeopathy

Homeopathy is probably the most controversial, complementary medical treatment today when it comes to being accepted or not by professionals in Western healthcare. The question whether homeopathy has any effect beyond placebo has been vigorously debated for the last 200 years. Homeopaths and their patients steadfastly claim that the method has positive effects, while many physicians maintain that it is all placebo. It is not easy to decide this matter since the method is very difficult to evaluate systematically and objectively. This is because homeopathic teachings are based on each patient being treated individually, and the therapy is made unique and personal for each patient. This makes it virtually impossible to conduct any studies on larger groups of patients, which means that the existing study results are of low quality and difficult to interpret. We will come back to these studies, but first, I would like to briefly describe the history and theory of homeopathy.

Homeopathy is based on a fundamental principle which states that *like cures like* or, in Latin, *similia similibus curentur*. This means that the same substance which creates symptoms of a disease in a healthy individual would also cure the disease in one who is ill. The word homeopathy is derived from the Greek *hómoios* (similar) and *páthos* (passion). The method was created in 1796 by German physician Samuel Hahnemann, and it was he who named it homeopathy. But the principle of like cures like is much older; it can be found in the teachings of Hippocrates, dating from the 5th century BCE and during the 17th century in the writings of Paracelsus (whom we met in the part about Bach flower remedies). Even the Romans believed in curing a disease with the same substance that caused it. I would like to point out that there is no scientific evidence whatsoever proving that this principle actually works.

According to one story (the truth of which is questionable), Hahnemann would have discovered the principle when he examined quinine by ingesting it. Supposedly, he was sceptical to the idea that the bark of the cinchona tree could cure malaria and he therefore ingested a piece of the bark to see what happened. The bark of the cinchona tree contains quinine, which is used to treat fever and malaria. Hahnemann experienced fever, shivering, and joint pain, which are all symptoms of malaria. He then concluded that substances which cause disease symptoms in healthy people will cure the disease in one who suffers from it. If this story is true, it is more likely that Hahnemann simply was allergic to quinine, which is a rather common allergy. Later researchers who have tried to create the same symptoms by ingesting cinchona bark have not felt anything.

During treatment, a patient is given homeopathic preparations designed to cure a disease using the same substance which causes it, only in much smaller concentrations. This dilution of the preparations, which is known as *potencialization* since it supposedly increases the *potency* of the preparations, is one of the most important principles in homeopathy. A substance is diluted with alcohol or distilled water and then shaken vigorously, supposedly activating the vital energies in the substance and thereby making it more potent. The principle has been debated by scientists who say that homeopathic preparations are diluted to such an extent that no molecules of the substance are left, rendering the preparations inert. Some homeopaths have claimed that there is something called "water memory," an ability that lets the water "remember" a substance that has been dissolved in it and transfer the properties of this substance to anyone drinking the water. Modern research has not been able to find any evidence of this water memory, but studies made with NMR cameras (nuclear magnetic resonance cameras) on dilutions have shown stable water structures. Researchers claim that this might be a sign of so-called supramolecular structures being able to exist even in dilutions that should not contain any active molecules. What do you think—does water have a "memory"?

Another key feature in homeopathy is *miasms*. Hahnemann claimed that certain diseases leave a residual injury or infection that he called a miasm (from the word *miasma*, a contagious power in Greek mythology). Hahnemann maintained that these miasms form when disease symptoms are relieved or supressed by conventional drugs without curing the underlying disease. The miasms would then cause chronic diseases. Critics claim that Hahnemann developed the theory of miasms causing chronic diseases because the homeopathic remedies failed to cure these diseases. Modern research in the fields of immunology and pathology have refuted the miasm theory.

Despite the massive criticism from scientists and physicians, homeopathy continues to be a popular treatment method, especially in Europe. The method has developed continuously and spread internationally, and is today popular also in North America and Asia. In recent years, there has been a sharp increase in the use of homeopathic remedies in India, where reports show that approximately 100 million people use only homeopathic medical care. However, the World Health Organization has made a statement that it does not support the use of homeopathy for the purpose of curing serious diseases such as malaria, tuberculosis and HIV.

As I mentioned earlier, there are plenty of studies that examine homeopathic preparations and their proposed effects on certain ailments. I would like to briefly present some of the results of these studies, but remember that the results are very uncertain.

One systematic overview indicates that the homeopathic medicine known as *Asafoetida* would be better than placebo for people with IBS and constipation. However, this study was performed in the 1970s when the reporting of trials was not as extensive as it is now, and it is therefore difficult to comment on the results.

One study containing 283 clinical trials examined whether homeopathy was effective against the inflammatory skin disease known as atopic dermatitis. The study yielded no clear results, but in most cases, no significant effects were seen.

Neither were any positive effects seen in the different studies that examined homeopathy as a treatment for headache and migraines, ADHD, sleep disorders and tinnitus. Studies on anxiety, depression and various pulmonary diseases have all been inconclusive, simply because the studies were too small.

Lastly, there are a number of studies indicating that homeopathy might have an analgesic effect in patients with fibromyalgia (a chronic pain condition, primarily affecting the muscles). However, these studies are also small or of poor quality.

The individual nature of the therapies and the use of preparations that do not contain any known molecules make it difficult to systematically study the effects of the treatments. However, those preparations that do contain active molecules (i.e. dilutions up to D-12) could be regarded as potential pharmaceuticals. Therefore, these preparations should be subjected to clinical studies and all the requirements that conventional pharmaceuticals are subjected to. Such studies should be able to prove an effect beyond placebo (or the opposite, i.e. that placebo is more effective), as well as pinpoint certain parameters regarding production and quality. But such rigorous studies are not performed on homeopathic preparations.

It is also difficult to study potential side effects from the preparations. But since the preparations are diluted to such an extent, it is unlikely that they would cause any serious adverse effects. However, there are reports of negative side effects, especially from homeopathic preparations in the areas of detox and weight loss. Given the current state of research and many health authorities' attitude towards homeopathy, I would advise against using the preparations for the treatment of all medical conditions where there is a better evidence-based alternative, at least before consulting your healthcare team.

Anthroposophic Medicine

The basic idea behind anthroposophy is similar to the philosophy of yoga, and anthroposophic remedies are made in a way that is similar to homeopathic preparations. Anthroposophy is often combined with other forms of therapy, which makes it difficult to isolate patient groups for clinical research.

The effects of anthroposophic medicine are just as difficult to discern as those of homeopathy or Bach flower remedies. However, their high level of dilution means that they are virtually harmless. As with other complementary methods, delayed care is the greatest risk with the use of anthroposophic medicine, if the practitioner lacks proper medical education.

Anthroposophic Medicine

Anthroposophy is a philosophy that was developed around 1913 by Austrian philosopher Rudolf Steiner. In short, the philosophy teaches that people can gain knowledge about the world as a whole by engaging actively in personal development, both physically and mentally. It is important to develop both the body and mind since the world is said to be divided into matter and spirit. The best way to personal growth includes a mix of personal observations, moral practice, work, meditation, and studies in the sciences and humanities. The word anthroposophy is derived from the Greek words *ántropos* (human) and *sofía* (wisdom). The anthroposophical movement comprises a number of different practical activities, such as Waldorf education, biodynamic agriculture, so called organic architecture, certain art movements and anthroposophic medicine. You can read all about anthroposophy in books and on the Internet, so we will only focus on the medical practice, which is counted among the complementary medical methods.

Anthroposophic medicine could just as well have fitted into the first chapter of this book, since it comprises both theoretical and practical tools borrowed from Eastern medical traditions—for example, meditation, Ayurveda, and physical exercises similar to qigong. But since homeopathic ideas and herbal remedies are also important elements I have chosen to place it here. Before we move on to the practical parts of anthroposophic medicine, I would like to describe the basic ideas behind the treatments.

Rudolf Steiner claimed that human beings are made up of four different substances or bodies:

- The physical body, which is connected to all physical matter, even minerals.
- The wave-shaped energy, which is also connected to physical matter. This energy is described as a force field or vitality that makes up the so called *ethereal body*. It is connected to each person's memory bank. Even animals and plants are said to have an ethereal body. It is this idea, that all living things are animate because they have an ethereal body that has led to anthroposophical influences on agricultural techniques, the environmental movement and biodynamic cultivation.
- The astral body, which has the ability to leave the physical body. That is what happens when we dream. Even animals are said to have an astral body, albeit not as complex as the human.
- The self, which leaves the body after death in order to be reborn. The belief in reincarnation is typical for both Hinduism and Buddhism, and anthroposophy has borrowed ideas from both of those religions.

Steiner claimed that spiritual experiences and characteristics may follow from one life to another. Diseases can do the same. Diseases can also arise from imbalances between the four substances/bodies, and the purpose of anthroposophic medicine is to achieve balance. Steiner also claimed that the human body lacks organs to observe the spiritual, but that there are latent spiritual organs in each person. Developing them is said to promote good health and personal growth. The development is achieved through three types of exercise: physical-spiritual, meditative, and moral exercises.

The physical-spiritual exercises consist of certain body movements. They are known as *eurhythmy*, and are somewhat similar to tai chi, qigong, and certain dances.

The meditative exercises aim to expand our consciousness. This may be achieved through meditation on something specific, immersion in certain texts or mantras, or focussing our attention on abstract objects such as geometric shapes. It is common to set aside some time each night for retrospection in order to feel satisfaction with the day.

There are six moral exercises:

- Concentration of thoughts – Thinking about a single specific thing for five minutes.
- Controlling the will – Performing an action that you have decided on, each day at a precise time.
- Emotional balance – Practising to refrain from uncontrolled outbursts of grief, joy, anger, and fear, since these seldom bring anything good.
- Positivity – Trying to see the good, valuable, and positive in everything.
- Openness – Trying to face the world without preconceptions and with open arms.
- Inner harmony – A summarising exercise where the goal is to achieve a harmonic balance between the qualities that have been practised in the previous exercises.

Anthroposophic remedies are manufactured in a way similar to homeopathic remedies, and it is thus equally difficult to tell if they are effective or not. It is also difficult to study anthroposophic medicine since it is comprised of several different therapies, both remedies and physical therapies, which in many cases are administered together. This makes it difficult to know which form of therapy gives the positive effect, or if it is the combination that does it. Furthermore, anthroposophic medicine is often used as complement to conventional pharmaceuticals and psychotherapy, which also makes it difficult to discern which treatment is effective. Most studies are small or show flaws in their methodology, which makes it even harder to analyse the results.

Having said this, I would like to highlight the fact that some people feel that anthroposophic medicine is helpful to them. Whether this is due to placebo or actual positive effects from the treatments is uncertain, but anthroposophic medicine is used in the treatment of depression, fatigue, headache and pain in the muscles and joints. It has also been tried against asthma, bronchitis, and influenza. A number of studies on animals have examined anthroposophic remedies containing different mistletoe extracts, and it has been shown that these extracts have immunomodulatory, cytotoxic, and antiviral properties. That a substance has cytotoxic properties means that it is toxic to cells, which means it could be used in chemotherapy. That is also the case in anthroposophic cancer treatments. However, these cytotoxic properties have not been confirmed in well-designed clinical studies. Nevertheless, the studies show that some patients experience an enhanced quality of life. In anthroposophic reports, these remedies have been administered together with other therapies, so it is difficult to tell which treatment was the effective one. Very few studies show any side effects from anthroposophic remedies.

The official healthcare system cannot recommend anthroposophic medicine until it has been proved that it has an effect beyond placebo. Furthermore, some experts are openly critical towards anthroposophy because a number of anthroposophists oppose the traditional vaccination programmes.

Before we leave the herbal medicines and move on to the world of the senses, I would like to give a few closing comments. A common argument for using health food and natural remedies rather than conventional chemically produced pharmaceuticals is that you will then escape the side effects from the drugs. Sure enough, conventional drugs have, as I mentioned in the introduction, side effects that may sound more or less horrific. But the *balance between beneficial effects and risk* is at least made very clear when it comes to these pharmaceuticals. That is not the case with natural remedies because they have not been through the same rigorous research and tests as the pharmaceuticals. My point is that you should not believe that all health food and natural remedies are harmless. Neither have their beneficial properties been proved in the same way as with conventional pharmaceuticals. If you want to know more about the most popular and best-selling natural remedies, I refer you to the book *Panacea*.

When it comes to Bach flower remedies, homeopathic, and anthroposophic remedies, it is highly unlikely that they are harmful if you purchase them from guaranteed safe retailers, such as authorised pharmacies. However, unauthorised and irresponsible marketing is widespread for products containing active chemical agents or even narcotics, with false promises that they only contain the stated homeopathic remedies. It is therefore very important that we as consumers stay informed and aware of the risks before we make a choice.

Healing Through the Senses

A number of the complementary medical treatments are based on stimulating the senses for therapeutic purposes. It is mainly the classical five senses (sight, hearing, taste, touch, and smell) that are stimulated, even though modern science recognises at least a couple more. The kinaesthetic sense, for example, lets us know the position of our body parts in relation to each other and to the surroundings. This way of sensing all parts of one's body has long been an important aspect of many Eastern treatment methods.

6 Healing Through the Senses

There are a number of complementary medical treatments that are based on stimulating the senses in order to promote healing. We are often taught that we have five senses: sight, hearing, taste, smell, and touch. Aristotle has already asserted as early as the 4th century BCE that these were the five senses of man. But today, researchers recognise at least a couple more. For example, we have the sense of balance, the kinaesthetic sense (which helps us perceive our own body and feeds information to the central nervous system about where each body part is), and the sense that registers pain. Nevertheless, within complementary medicine, it is still mainly the "classical" five senses that are stimulated for therapeutic purposes.

However, it is interesting to highlight the kinaesthetic sense, which is not very well known outside the scientific community. This sense is also known as proprioception, a Latin term which literally means "individual grasp," which is the body's own way of sensing the position of each body part. It is a very useful sense. Just imagine: if we did not always know, more or less unconsciously, where our body parts were in relation to each other and to the surroundings, it would be very difficult to move or even perform the simplest of everyday tasks. When the police try to determine whether a driver is intoxicated, they sometimes use proprioception. Normally, a person can close their eyes and put their finger on the tip of their nose, since the body's kinaesthetic sense tells us where the finger and the nose are in relation to each other. This sense is numbed in an intoxicated person, making it much more difficult for them to find the spot. From a complementary medical point of view, the kinaesthetic sense is primarily interesting because it is connected with our life energy, that is, our qi or prana. When you close your eyes and concentrate on, let us say, your hand—can you "feel" it? You may feel a slight tingle in your hand, you sense it without seeing it or moving it. This way of perceiving all parts of your body is important in many Eastern philosophies, and it is based on perceiving the energy that flows through the body. Western researchers would probably rather tell you that we are dealing with proprioception, but is there really that much of a difference?

Chromotherapy

Despite a long tradition, there are no research results providing evidence for the claims that colours can affect our wellbeing and health, or that the human body would emit an aura of any physiological significance. The colours that we can see are electromagnetic radiation within a specific range of wavelengths, which we call visible light. When the light reflects off different surfaces, we perceive different colours. However, the claims related to how colours can affect our mood might be true to a certain degree.

Chromotherapy

Chromotherapy, or colour therapy, is not actually based on stimulating our sense of sight but since we perceive colours through our eyes, and since chromotherapy uses decorative elements that are meant to be experienced through sight, I have chosen to place chromotherapy in this chapter. The basis of chromotherapy is the idea that different colours consist of energy waves which affect us both physically and mentally in different ways. It is said that all living matter, including humans, emits certain vibrations. The frequency of these vibrations reflects our health condition by indicating balance or imbalance. Chromotherapy can be regarded as a kind of "frequency medicine," where the energy waves of the different colours are said to help balance the body's inherent vibrations. Each human being is surrounded by an energy field, an aura, that is said to consist of several vibrating fields. A healthy person emits a balanced and intense colour field similar to the spectrum of the rainbow. The different colours in the aura are considered to be related to different personality traits. In order to determine which treatment is needed, the aura is examined, as well as the colour of the tongue, eyes, and lips. Sometimes, psychological tests are used in which the therapist examines which colours the patient prefers. After having determined which colours/vibrations are missing, treatment is given using certain means such as:

- Offering water and various foods that have been treated with different colours;
- Decorating one's surroundings (clothes, bedding, curtains, carpets, lights, etc.);
- Offering crystals and salts;
- Using coloured cards and lamps; and
- Mentally evoking colours and shapes, for example through meditation and visualisation techniques. You may, for example, be asked to imagine that the air you breathe is a certain colour (this is more common in treatments that also involve the seven most important chakras in the body and the colours associated with each; see Chapter 1 for more information about chakras).

Chromotherapy has a long history: in ancient Egypt, coloured minerals, rocks, crystals, ointments, and dyes were used as remedies. Colours were also used in a variety of therapeutic ways in East Asia and ancient Persia. During the Middle Ages in Europe, Paracelsus advocated light and colour therapy to restore good health. In the West, chromotherapy became popular in the 20th century when the founder of anthroposophy, Rudolf Steiner, developed Goethe's colour theory and applied it to medicine.

Despite the long tradition, there is no evidence-based research supporting the claims that chromotherapy can affect our wellbeing and our health, nor that there is an "aura" of any physiological significance emanating from the human body. The colours we humans can see are really electromagnetic radiation within a specific range of wavelengths that we call visible light. We cannot actually see this light either; what we perceive as colours is the radiation as it reflects off different surfaces. The surfaces then appear to be of distinct colours. However, the idea that different colours have different qualities and affect us differently is widespread, and some of the claims may be partly true. For example, it seems like rooms painted in red or yellow tones have an invigorating effect while rooms painted green or blue have a calming effect. It is often said that "cold" colours like blue and green can make you feel colder than "warm" colours like red and yellow. However, it seems the intensity of the colour is more important than the actual colour. Below are listed some of the qualities that different colours are said to be associated with, as well as their proposed healing effects. Light shades are said to have a stronger healing effect than darker shades.

- Red – Courage, liberation, passion, excitement, expansion. Softens up stiff muscles and joints.
- Orange – Self-confidence, practical knowledge, action. Relieves intestinal cramps.
- Yellow – Intellect, awareness, self-confidence, self-esteem. Removes toxins; promotes weight loss.
- Green – Harmony, stability, clarity, understanding, economic success. Important healing colour.
- Blue – Wisdom, truth, intelligence, calmness, creativity. Used against stiff neck, thyroid problems, unwillingness to speak out.
- Indigo – Strength, power, the ability to see and unravel obscurity. Painkiller.
- Purple – Peace, spirituality, visions. Used against headaches, internal inflammations. Also said to provide insight when solving conflicts.
- Black – Abundance. Strengthens self-discipline.
- White – Pure state, trust. Contains an equal amount of all colours.
- Gold – Faith, unity, self-knowledge. Relieves irritated colon and underactive thyroid gland.
- Silver – Associated with the cosmic intelligence. Subdues emotions, purifies the body.
- Turquoise – Goal oriented, promotes soul-searching and understanding of the self.
- Grey – Optimism (light grey is said to be calming).

So-called visible light is only a fraction of the electromagnetic spectrum, which extends from radio waves with very long wavelengths to gamma radiation with very short wavelengths (see picture). The entire electromagnetic spectrum, including visible light, affects us in different ways. Just think of how we use X-rays in hospitals, how harmful radioactive gamma radiation is, or how the sun's ultraviolet radiation can give us a nice tan. It is therefore not so farfetched to think that visible light, divided into the distinct colours that we perceive, can affect us in various ways. What do you think?

Light Therapy

Light therapy rooms are often equipped with so-called light boxes which simulate daylight and are 10 times stronger than the average office light. It is common to stay in the room for one to two hours. It is mainly autumn and winter depressions that are supposed to be treated with this method. It has not yet been proved whether this therapy method has any effect beyond placebo.

Light Therapy

Light therapy is a collective term denoting various treatment methods where light is used for therapeutic purposes. Some of them, such as photodynamic therapy (PDT), are clinically useful treatment methods, usually for different types of skin diseases or certain cancers. However, when we talk of light therapy in complementary medicine, we usually mean a form of therapy where bright light is used to treat autumn and winter depressions said to be due to the lack of light during the dark seasons. It is not uncommon for spa facilities and other health institutions to have a light therapy room. In Sweden, there are also light rooms in several hospitals. Certain spa facilities also have a room for "darkness therapy," where you get to rest in a dark room, usually to soothing music or sounds in headphones. Apart from the darkness, it is difficult to tell what makes darkness therapy different from certain other relaxation techniques, and so I choose to not describe it in any detail.

Light therapy rooms are often equipped with so-called light boxes which simulate daylight and are approximately 10 times stronger than the average office light. A typical light therapy session has you spend between one and two hours in the light room. Light therapy is also said to be effective if your diurnal rhythm has been disturbed for some reason. It has not yet been proved whether the form of light therapy described here has any effect beyond placebo.

Image Therapy

Various forms of image therapy have been used for thousands of years. Today, it is used in several areas on an individual level and in group therapy, as well as in the treatment of trauma and PTSD, to relieve anxiety and depression, and to provide increased quality of life for cancer patients. There are ongoing studies examining treatment of chronic pain conditions.

The studies that have been conducted as of today are small and suffer from flaws in methodology, so no general recommendations can be given. However, no negative side effects have been seen from the treatments.

Image Therapy

Image therapy is a collective term denoting a number of treatment methods where the creation of images is used to express and communicate emotions and thoughts. Artistic techniques like drawing, painting, and sculpture are combined with reflective dialogue and various forms of psychotherapy such as Guided Imagery. The idea is that both the creative process and the dialogue related to the image created have therapeutic value. Using materials, tools, and techniques is also considered to provide sensory experiences and make you aware of memories.

Both complex connections and different time perspectives can be expressed simultaneously in an image. The language of images is circular, as opposed to verbal language, which is linear. The image therapist provides all necessary materials, a place to work in, guidelines for the work, his/her time and attention, and he/she will also support the client's creative expression. The method is aimed both at people who, for various reasons, have not mastered the verbal language or who lack words to express emotions, and at people who are overly verbal or tend to intellectualise. Creating images provides structure, which facilitates verbalisation and develops the ability to use symbols. The creative process promotes learning by activating the whole brain, both the right and left hemispheres. Image therapy has also been shown to reduce symptoms related to pain and anxiety.

Various forms of image therapy have been used for millennia and their therapeutic value has been recognised for a long time. Image therapy was further developed during the 1940s in Europe and the United States, in connection with the rehabilitation of war victims, especially children who had experienced traumatising events. Image therapy has been used in Sweden since the 1960s, and today, it is used in several areas, on an individual level as well as in group and family therapy, in the treatment of trauma and PTSD (post-traumatic stress disorder).

Studies indicate that Guided Imagery could have positive effects on mobility and quality of life for people with arthrosis and Parkinson's disease. Image therapy also seems to increase the quality of life for people with various cancers. Other studies show that image therapy reduces anxiety and depression and increases self-esteem. According to one study, it also seems to help pregnant women with anxiety. Ongoing studies are examining the use of two other forms of image therapy, motor imagery and mirror therapy, in the treatment of chronic pain. However, most of the studies that have been conducted on image therapy so far are rather small and often show some flaws in methodology, so the healthcare system cannot give any general recommendations regarding image therapy. No side effects have been observed from any of the treatment methods, though.

Sound Therapy

The idea behind sound therapy is that each cell, tissue, and organ in our bodies has its own vibration frequency. Resonance can be achieved through sound waves of the same frequency as the organ and a certain physiological/therapeutic effect can be registered. Sound healing is a way to "tune" different parts of the body to the "correct frequency," using certain tools such as a tuning fork, resonance bowl, gong, crystal bowl, or simply the voice of the therapist.

There is no scientific evidence supporting the use of either music or sound healing in this way. There are, however, studies indicating that sound can affect heart frequency.

Sound Therapy

Sound therapy is a collective term denoting several different treatment methods where sounds or music is used in various ways. One such method is music therapy, which has developed rapidly in the last decades, and into which a great deal of research has been done. Studies suggest positive effects on both mental and physical ailments. Among other things, it has been shown that heart rate and blood pressure can be affected by listening to music, which can be used to treat different cardiovascular diseases. Other ailments on which music therapy seems to have an effect include schizophrenia, dementia, Alzheimer's, Parkinson's disease, depression, and Tourette's syndrome. Internationally, Norway is an important country for both research and practice in music therapy. Two major research centres are located there, where several different therapy methods are used and evaluated. Music therapy is also used in social work at medical clinics, retirement homes, and in prisons.

Another form of sound therapy is known as music acupuncture. The idea behind this method is that each cell, tissue and organ in our bodies has its own vibration frequency (similar ideas are expressed in chromotherapy and crystal healing). If you know the frequency of a particular organ, you can reach it by using sound waves of the same frequency. Resonance occurs and the effect resembles a deep massage at the molecular level. This supposedly reduces stress and resolves blockages, which brings balance and harmony to the organ being massaged. There is no scientific evidence that music acupuncture would work in this manner, but, as I stated above, there are studies indicating that sound can affect at least the heart rate.

A similar theory is the basis of what we may call sound healing. The idea is that imbalances in the body cause it to go "out of tune". This in turn causes blockages that can be bad for our health. Sound healing supposedly helps "tune" the body to the right frequency. Tools for this include tuning forks, resonance bowls, gongs, crystal bowls, or simply the therapist's voice. There is no scientific evidence supporting this form of sound therapy either.

Two types of sound therapy are used specifically to alleviate tinnitus problems. One is called tinnitus masking, and it is based on the idea of adding more sounds, for example a neutral soughing sound, to mask the tinnitus sounds. The other is called TRT (*Tinnitus Retraining Therapy*), and it is a combination of cognitive behavioural therapy and neurological music therapy. The idea is to train the brain to better manage the tinnitus, or even filter it out. Both therapy methods aim to alleviate tinnitus problems, not cure the tinnitus. If you can focus less on your tinnitus, it is easier to relax and hopefully you will escape many of the problems associated with tinnitus, such as stress. Since tinnitus is a subjective experience, and we lack an objective way of measuring it, it is difficult to objectively measure whether these therapies work. One study shows that TRT is more effective than tinnitus masking, but no general conclusions can be drawn due to the low quality of the study. In the United States, research is being done on TRT treatment for members of the Armed Forces with tinnitus.

Aroma Therapy

Aroma therapy uses scented essential oils said to have healing properties. Essential oils exist naturally in different plants, from trees and bushes to flowers, and they can be extracted through pressing or distillation. Among the more common essential oils are rose oil, almond oil, and bergamot oil. The oils are used in the manufacture of perfumes or as flavouring in food, but also for therapeutic purposes. Considering that the oils come from plants, one could regard aroma therapy as a specific branch of herbal medicine, but since it is mainly via our sense of smell that the therapy is received, I chose to place it in this chapter.

During an aroma therapy session, the essential oils are heated in certain aroma lamps before being inhaled. They can also be applied directly to the skin through massage or given in a bath. Aroma therapy can also be combined with other methods of complementary medicine, such as yoga. During an aroma yoga session, you perform yoga exercises while simultaneously applying essential oils.

Aroma therapy is a very old treatment method, described in sources from ancient Egypt and dated to around 3,500 BCE. It has a long tradition in other cultures as well. When the distillation process was developed in the Middle Ages, essential oils became even more popular as medicine and perfume. During World War II, French surgeon Jean Valnet became a pioneer as he used essential oils as a germicide when working on wounded soldiers. This prompted further development of aroma therapy in France and the UK.

Aroma therapy is mainly given for the purpose of relieving stress, but in 1993, physicians at Queen Elizabeth Psychiatric Hospital in Birmingham in the UK reported that epileptic patients did not suffer as many seizures when they used essential oils. A study was conducted the year after at Middlesex Hospital in London, and it showed that aroma therapy had a calming effect in heart patients. Aroma therapy is often used in England in hospices and palliative care.

Researchers are unsure of what makes aroma therapy effective, but there are three theories that may explain the effects. The first theory is that the smell of the oils primarily affects our sense of smell and that these smells can awaken memories and emotions. If so, they might also stimulate the nervous system and the glands that produce and release hormones. This might explain why the oils relieve stress. The second theory is that oil molecules penetrate the skin and cleanse mucous membranes in the throat and airways. If the molecules penetrate all the way to the blood, they might also affect the cell membranes. The third theory is that the oils' antiseptic and anti-inflammatory properties are beneficial for our health and strengthen the immune system. Whatever the reason, aroma therapy is effective against certain ailments. However, I want to point out that some side effects have been reported, including heart rhythm disturbance, vomiting, hypertension, erythema, dizziness, fainting, sleep disorders, itching, allergic reactions, and acid-base imbalance (imbalance in the blood pH). Therefore, you should consult your healthcare team before trying aroma therapy.

> **Tactile Massage**
>
> Tactile massage is said to provide increased wellbeing by stimulating the release of the hormone oxytocin, which is related to community, trust, care, parental emotions, reduced aggressiveness, and anxiety. However, researchers have not yet been able to determine whether this massage really releases the hormone.
>
> Today, tactile massage is used in prenatal and palliative care, as well as a few other areas.

Tactile Massage

Tactile massage can be said to be "healthcare through touching." The tactile sense is our sense of touch. It is located mainly in the skin layer known as dermis (or corium) and contains receptors sensitive to touch, pressure, vibration, heat, and cold. Tactile massage is a relatively new form of massage that originates in Sweden. Touch is applied with a soft, even pressure and tactile massage is thus different from regular massage where you knead and work the muscles. Since this method is rather new, researchers have not yet had the time to study its effects. Those who maintain that tactile massage works, state that it provides pain relief, relaxation, and increased wellbeing by stimulating secretion of the hormone oxytocin. This hormone is connected with community, trust, care, parental emotions, reduced aggressiveness, and reduced anxiety, so if tactile massage really helps in the secretion of oxytocin, it is possible that it has the mentioned effects. However, researchers are still uncertain whether the massage actually releases oxytocin. Today, tactile massage is used in prenatal and palliative care. It is also said to be effective against depression in elderly people who have lost their partner, i.e. people used to being touched and now lacking it.

Aside from the treatment methods mentioned above, there are many more forms of treatment that allegedly stimulate the senses for therapeutic purposes.

However, those reviewed here are the most common. They all have two things in common: their therapeutic effects have not been sufficiently proved and, generally speaking, they have no side effects. That means that if you feel like trying any of them, in most cases there is no risk involved – but it is always a good idea to consult your healthcare team first, especially if you have a medical condition or use any medicines. We will now move on to the last section of this book, which deals with physical exercise.

Healing Through Motion

Two treatment methods are based on the idea that humans are built to move and also benefit from it. Dance therapy is a complementary medical method. Physical activity is an evidence-based complement, and sometimes even an alternative, to conventional treatments.

7 Healing Through Motion

We will now go from healing through our senses to healing through motion. In this last chapter, we will begin by reviewing one additional method of complementary medicine: dance therapy. We will then move on to a form of treatment that is now being regarded as an evidence-based complement to, and in some cases even as an alternative to, certain pharmaceuticals: physical activity. As I stated in the beginning of the book, there must be evidence-based research supporting a treatment method before the public healthcare system can recommend it. When it comes to physical activity, a great many studies clearly show the health benefits of exercise, both for physical and mental wellbeing, as well as for preventive purposes. Today, you can even get PAP, physical activity on prescription. We will briefly review the historical research on physical activity and also take a closer look at a few ailments on which physical activity has positive effects. But first, I would like to describe a form of therapy where movement and dance are used in a special way.

Dance Therapy

Dance therapy is based primarily on the idea that body and soul interact, both consciously and unconsciously. Movement is said to have a symbolic function that can contribute to increased awareness of the soul. Dance therapy is said to work well for people with mental or psychosomatic problems or for people who need to process crises or unresolved conflicts.

Studies indicate that dance therapy can lead to improvement in walking for patients with Parkinson's disease. It also seems to relieve anxiety and improve balance, mental health, and quality of life. It has also proved effective against obesity. Dance therapy can also be regarded as a preventive health and fitness activity, and it may bring more inspiration and joy to one's life.

Dance Therapy

Dance therapy is an artistic form of therapy that includes dancing and movement, images, and the spoken word. Important elements include communication and processes on a non-verbal level, i.e. you express emotions through gestures and movement instead of words. One of the goals of dance therapy is to increase our physical, emotional, and mental presence in order to make us more aware of what goes on inside of us and in our interactions with other people. Thus, mindfulness is often a part of dance therapy, both in stillness and in movement. The anthroposophical movement therapy known as eurhythmy is somewhat reminiscent of dance therapy.

In the beginning, dance therapy was considered a form of healing, but it has evolved and is now regarded as a form of psychotherapy. Dance as therapy emerged during the 1940s in America and is now an established form of therapy worldwide. In Europe, dance and movement therapy have existed as treatment methods for a number of decades, and there are regulated dance therapy education classes based in modern psychodynamic theories, with elements of cognitive behavioural therapy.

Researchers have not been able to prove exactly what it is in dance therapy that creates the positive effects, except that it is a form of treatment based on physical activity, which is always good. The American Dance Therapy Association (ADTA) defines dance and movement therapy as "the psychotherapeutic use of movement to further the emotional, cognitive, physical and social integration of the individual." It is assumed that the body, mind, and soul are linked and that movement and emotions are constantly influencing each other. It is therefore also assumed that your emotions can be influenced by certain physical movements. The dancing and movement are supposed to set free and create certain moods that in turn create joy and lead to improved quality of life and better health.

Thus, dance therapy is mainly based on the belief that the body and soul interact, both consciously and unconsciously. Movement is regarded as having a symbolic function that may contribute to increased awareness of the soul. It is said that dance therapy may help people with psychological or psychosomatic problems, such as sleep disorders, anxiety, pain, tension, and eating disorders, as well as for people who need to process unresolved conflicts. For people who are in some form of crisis in life, dance therapy may be a way to process the crisis. Dancing can also be used as a preventive health and fitness activity, or by anyone looking for more inspiration and joy in life.

The majority of studies on dance therapy describe the positive effects it seems to have, but the results should be taken with caution since most of the studies are small and of inferior quality. Some studies suggest that dance therapy may lead to an improvement in walking for people with Parkinson's disease. It also seems to relieve anxiety and improve balance, mental health, and quality of life. Since it is a form of therapy based on physical activity, it has proved effective against obesity. Ongoing research is looking into whether dance therapy can be effective against dementia.

When it comes to negative side effects of dance therapy, it should be regarded as any other physical activity. Relatively few negative side effects have been reported, in view of the large number of participants around the world. The most common reported negative side effects include muscle strains, ligament injuries and sprains.

Physical Activity

Physical activity is a very effective measure for improving general health. It retards or prevents cardiovascular diseases, high blood pressure, colon cancer, diabetes, osteoarthritis, osteoporosis, chronic pain, obesity, and mental disorders. It also improves health for people who suffer from conditions such as MS, stroke, COPD, autism, etc.

The side effect profile of physical activity is far better than for most drugs.

Physical activity is good for humans, from the cellular level to mental well-being. If you train on a level appropriate to your conditions, there are practically no risks.

The Eastern training philosophies yoga, vyayam, Tibetan rites, qigong, and tai chi are also based on physical activity and thus might be effective. The evidence-based healthcare system still finds it difficult to recommend them. This is because of the underlying theory of a life energy within each of us that we have to balance using physical and mental exercises. Researchers have not yet been able to measure any such energy, and so they can neither confirm nor rule out its existence.

Physical Activity

Movement and physical activity have always been part of human life. We have walked, run, jumped, and climbed for as long as we have existed. In fact, it is movement that separates humans and animals from plants. The most important function of the brain is to make sure that we can move; it is the lack of a brain that is the major reason why plants cannot move in the usual sense. In simpler organisms, the brain might even lose its function if the organism stops moving. One example of this is the ascidian, or sea squirt, whose life is divided into two phases. It is born a larva and spends most of its time in search of a place where it can settle. Once it has found a nice spot, it attaches to it and "eats up" its brain. This is done to conserve energy. The brain is the most energy-consuming organ in the body, and since the ascidian will not have to move around anymore once it has attached itself, it simply has no need for a brain.

Now, why do I mention this? Well, this example clearly shows the connection between the function of the brain in vertebrates and physical activity. If we do not move, it is not only our muscles that wither away—the brain also needs exercise. Now, do not be alarmed; your brain will not wither away just because you spend a lot of time sitting down; what I mean here is that it seems pretty obvious that we humans are made to move, and that it would also be bad for us to not be physically active. But in order for the healthcare system and the government to recommend physical activity, they need evidence-based research, and that has taken quite a while to collect. But now we have it.

We humans have a basic need for a natural cycle of activity followed by rest. This cycle developed during the Stone Age, when the days were filled with hunting, gathering, and other activities, and people slept during the dark hours. This so-called Palaeolithic cycle ("Stone Age cycle") reminds us of today's recommendations to the public; with our sedentary lifestyle and welfare diseases, the recommendation is "back to basic." Later on—around 10,000 BCE—when we began to farm the land and specialise in less physically demanding work than constant hunting, healers and shamans began to emphasise the importance of physical activity. They suggested that a long and healthy life is based on preventing ill health through proper diet and physical activity. Similar recommendations can be found in early written sources, such as in the most important book of Traditional Chinese Medicine, "The Yellow Emperor's Classic of Internal Medicine," and in early Indian Ayurvedic texts. These texts were, as we have seen, important to the development of qigong, tai chi, yoga, vyayam, and similar philosophies in which physical exercise plays a major role. In Europe, it is mainly physicians and philosophers in ancient Greece, who have most influenced the idea of physical activity as a way to prevent ill health. The "Father of Modern Medicine," Hippocrates, as well as Herodicus and Galen, studied what was then called physiotherapy and advocated an active lifestyle with lots of exercise and training.

Modern physiological studies were first conducted in the 1770s by researchers like Antoine Lavoisier and Pierre de Laplace. They used techniques that let them measure people's oxygen absorption and carbon dioxide production, during both rest and exercise. During the 20th century, researchers made great breakthroughs. One example is a study from 1927 in which it was first proved that endurance training improves the effectiveness of the cardiovascular system. This study was followed by several others that examined the connection between physical activity and cholesterol metabolism. We have since seen a vast number of studies verifying many of the positive results and proving that physical activity can be related to health.

Surely, it must seem quite clear that the physical treatment and training methods that we reviewed in Chapter 1—yoga, vyayam, Tibetan rites, qigong, and tai chi—are effective because they are based on physical activity. But if so, why is it so difficult for our evidence-based healthcare system to recommend them? The answer is the underlying theories. Evidence-based research and healthcare cannot accept the idea that there is an energy body, qi energy, or prana, within us that we balance by performing various physical and mental exercises—at least not until this energy has been measured and quantified. But if people believe in this energy, and that belief induces them to engage in physical activity, that is a good thing, right? What do you think? And even if this energy does not exist, then even a placebo, as we have seen, can be an effective part of a healing process.

Modern research on physical activity and its effect on our health has come to one general conclusion: physical activity is a very effective measure for improving general health, reducing mortality, retarding or preventing cardiovascular disease, hypertension, colon cancer, diabetes, osteoarthritis, osteoporosis, chronic pain, obesity, mental disorders, etc. Studies also suggest that physical activity:

- Can improve physical performance and muscle strength in people who have suffered some form of spinal cord injury;
- Gives better strength, balance, and stability in the elderly, and reduces the risk of dementia;

- Improves motor and social skills in people with autism;
- Strengthens the muscles of people with MS;
- Improves rehabilitation after a stroke; and
- Increases the physical capacity and oxygen absorption of people with asthma or chronic obstructive pulmonary disease (COPD).

It has been observed that physical activity performed over longer and successive periods stimulates most of the body's different organ systems in a health-promoting manner. The musculoskeletal system—that is, skeleton, tissues, joints, ligaments, and muscles—undergoes a positive change, and so does the heart muscle. Tendons are strengthened, and muscle mass increases, which helps to retard or prevent osteoporosis. The number of capillaries increases, resulting in a better flow of blood and nutrients. As muscle capacity increases, and the HPA axis (a system of hormonal glands responsible for the body's stress hormones) is positively affected, blood pressure is lowered. The increased flow of blood to the lungs strengthens the respiratory system. Positive changes also occur in the body's metabolism; for example, mitochondria increase in size and number (which helps the cells in energy production), myoglobin content increases (which also benefits the cells), and glycogen storage increases (which helps us to better store carbohydrates). In addition, the use of other forms of energy, such as free fatty acids from the body's various depots, increases, improving the lipid profile (which refers to blood fats, cholesterol and weight). The positive stress that the body is exposed to at moderate levels of exercise supports the function of the immune system, which leads to a reduction of certain infections and cancers. If you are interested in the connection between physical activity and the brain, there are lots of good books out there about the positive effects that exercise has on our brain functions.

I would also like to state that the side effect profile of physical activity is far better than for most drugs. During light to medium exercise, the risk of adverse effects is almost non-existent. The risk of injury increases if you intensify the exercise without being physically ready for it. That is why it is important to train at the proper level, and there are many good trainers who can help you with this. However, if you have a medical condition, run a higher risk of cardiovascular disease, or are unused to exercise, you should consult your medical team before you begin an intensive training program. But you can begin immediately with simpler physical activities! Today's recommendations state that adults should be physically active at least half an hour a day, but that is a low minimum. If you can exercise more, then do it. Go for a brisk walk, do some gardening, play sports, take the bike to work, the stairs instead of the elevator—whatever suits you best. If your work is a sedentary one, it is important that you stand up and move your body now and then. Try walking around your desk a couple of times every hour. Or why not try office yoga? Public health authorities usually list the recommendations for physical activity on their websites.

To conclude this chapter, we can say that physical activity is good for us, from the cellular level to our mental health, and if you train on a level appropriate to your state, there are practically no risks. Can there be a better medicine?

In the next chapter, we finish the book with a discussion about the gap between the public healthcare system and complementary medicine. I also put forward a few ideas about the potential integration of complementary medicine into the public healthcare system. But first, I would like to tie the book's main ideas together into a short reflection about balance. I have talked a lot about balance in this book, especially balance between the physical body and the energy body that many Eastern philosophies say is a part of us humans. To many people in the Western world, especially in healthcare and the scientific community, it can be a leap of faith to embrace that idea. But to strive for balance is something that all of us can do. Finding the balance between what you eat, how you think, what activities you engage in, and how personally adapted but actively you live is perhaps the key to a longer life—or at least a more fulfilling one.

Conclusion

Mending a Divided Healthcare SystemAround 80 percent of the world's population is treated using methods outside the evidence-based healthcare system. At the same time, the future of evidence-based healthcare is characterised by high-tech solutions, standardisation, and economic interests.

Despite the fact that consumers continue to use unknown preparations and treatments without any proven effect, very few resources are granted to researching complementary medicine.

Consumers turn to "experts" in complementary medicine, who often lack essential knowledge of the human body's pathophysiological processes.

Integrating certain complementary medical methods into the official healthcare system could help us avoid the risk for complications from delayed care and incorrect diagnoses. It would also make it easier for researchers to study these methods and their potential effects.

Conclusion
Mending a Divided Healthcare System

Today, the most common view of complementary medical treatments is that they are alternatives to official healthcare, that they exist outside it, and are separated from it by an abyss that is very difficult to bridge. On one side of this abyss are physicians, researchers, and the entire evidence-based healthcare machine with the pharmaceutical companies at the head. On the other side are therapists and practitioners, treated people, instructors, and theoreticians along with thousands of years of experience. The problem, if you choose to regard it as such, is that more and more people gather on the side of complementary medicine. The interest in treatments that are not based on conventional drugs grows by the day. Globally, evidence-based healthcare is at a disadvantage: as I mentioned in Chapter 5, around 80 percent of the world's population is treated with methods outside the evidence-based system. These treatments mainly consist of herbal remedies, various forms of shamanism and healing, traditional-based medicine, and individual therapies. At the same time, the future of evidence-based healthcare seems characterised by high-tech solutions, standardisation, and economic interests.

As we have seen, many of the complementary medical treatments base their proposed effects on something other than active substances, chemical molecules and other things which evidence-based research can measure and quantify. That is why researchers have failed to present a logical and consistent model of explanation, and so they reject most complementary methods. The fact that experience speaks for these methods and that people feel they benefit from them is deemed inconsequential. The attitude seems to be: if we do not know how, if we cannot explain why, we reject the hypothesis, and call the inexplicable effect placebo. Why keep on researching when we already know everything, when our principles are firm and unwavering?

In view of how we have constantly had to revise our "truths" throughout history when new discoveries were made, this attitude is incomprehensible to me. Thankfully, not all researchers reject the complementary methods or the placebo effect. On the contrary, the interest among researchers in complementary medicine and the placebo effect has grown in recent years, and some studies in the field are hopeful. The problem is that several of the publications on complementary medicine that can be found in scientific periodicals fail to fulfil the most basic requirements to be regarded as "valid medical research." That is why we need more large-scale and well-structured studies. Only when the studies fulfil the requirements that evidence-based science has put up can the results be taken seriously by "the other side." Until then, advocates of solely evidence-based healthcare have an excuse to not listen. You could also look at it this way: if you cannot prove a physical effect from the complementary methods, you must at least prove that they could form a complement that benefits some patient groups, and clarify which specific groups are benefitted and under what circumstances.

However, for those who wish to research complementary medicine, it can be difficult to receive the necessary grants to finance the research. Despite the fact that consumers continue to use "unknown preparations" and treatments that lack a proven effect, our universities, research centres, and experts choose to spend neither time nor money on researching complementary medicine. Consumers and patients then turn to "experts," who often lack essential knowledge of the human body's pathophysiological processes. Despite the best intentions, these therapists may risk their patients' health and delay proper care. It is my opinion that this is an unsustainable and highly dangerous situation that can lead to suffering and ill health. It is a serious health hazard that our current healthcare could well be accused of and condemned for in the future.

I would like to point out that both sides have their flaws. There is great nonchalance among self-proclaimed experts on both sides. To say that it has been proved that complementary methods have no value to consumers, and that they are only "dangerous" is just as irresponsible and nonchalant as promising cure and relief in an unfounded manner. Neither side seems to have enough knowledge of the other side's commitment to have a substantial basis for their claims. This phenomenon is prevalent is most healthcare systems in the Western world.

How, then, can we bridge the abyss between evidence-based healthcare and complementary medicine? One possible solution is to integrate some of the complementary methods in a controlled manner into the official healthcare system. In this way, trained medical personnel can assist those interested in treating themselves or in getting in touch with the proper healthcare providers. This would mean avoiding one of the greatest risks associated with the use of complementary medicine, which is complications due to delayed care and faulty diagnoses. Should complementary medicine be integrated into the official healthcare system, it would also make it easier for researchers to study the different methods and their effectiveness. However, whether the already overburdened primary care system can undertake this task needs to be further evaluated. As I mentioned earlier, some of the methods have already been integrated into the system, and others are well on their way in. Acupuncture and qigong can be recommended, certain health foods are advocated by some physicians, and physical activity can be given on prescription. It is a start, but we can go so much farther—provided the will to do so exists.

If complementary medicine is to be integrated into the official healthcare system, it has to start at the university level. Students of medicine must be trained in complementary methods. This may be a problem since pharmaceutical companies often give financial support to medical universities around the world, and these companies are probably not very interested in students learning methods that which would deprive them of income. But if complementary medicine were to find its way into medical studies, it could have some very interesting results. If the students were willing to face "the world of energy" with their own perceptive abilities and not primarily with their intellect, it might upset the entire paradigm. Perhaps our body, health, and healthcare are something other than what our scientists are convinced of. Perhaps we will look differently on the processes of disease and recovery in the future. What do you think?

Regardless of whether this is the future or not, it is a fact today that many of the complementary treatment methods are appreciated by a significant number of consumers and that the interest continues to grow. However, as long as the complementary methods lie outside the official healthcare system, no general recommendations can be given, neither for nor against, and it is completely up to you as an individual if you want to try them or not. But entering the world of complementary medicine as a consumer is not easy. Misleading information, delayed diagnoses, and marketing of harmful or ineffective preparations have caused complementary medicine to be stamped as a health hazard instead of the resource that it could be. As a consumer, you need unbiased information, knowledge, and perhaps some guidance to find your way. It is my hope that this book has provided you with some insight into the world of complementary medicine.

www.ingramcontent.com/pod-product-compliance
Lightning Source LLC
Chambersburg PA
CBHW061511180526
45171CB00001B/138